G000128856

Adam's Burden

Adam's Burden

An Explorer's Personal Odyssey Through Prostate Cancer

Charles Neider

MADISON BOOKS
Lanham • New York • Oxford

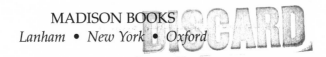

First Madison Books edition 2001

This Madison Books hardcover edition of *Adam's Burden* is an original publication.
It is published by arrangement with the author.

Published by Madison Books
4720 Boston Way
Lanham, Maryland 20706

12 Hid's Copse Road
Cumnor Hill, Oxford OX2 9JJ, England

Distributed by National Book Network

Library of Congress Cataloging-in-Publication Data

Neider, Charles, 1915-
   Adam's burden : an explorer's personal odyssey through prostate cancer / Charles Neider.
     p. cm.
   ISBN 1-56833-239-4 (cloth : alk. paper)
   1. Neider, Charles, 1915—Health. 2. Prostate—Cancer—Patients—United
States—Biography. I. Title.

RC280.P7 N45 2001
362.1'9699463—dc21
[B]
                                                   2001041048

To Edward M. Soffen

Contents

Preface

There is currently what some people consider to be an epidemic of prostate cancer, of unknown cause, in the United States. Since 1973 the incidence of this disease has risen by 30 percent. It is not generally agreed to what extent the rise is due to our increasing ability to detect this cancer. The most common cancer among American men, it is second to lung cancer as a cause of cancer deaths in the United States. Each year more than 150,000 men in the United States are diagnosed with prostate cancer. Some 35,000 Americans were expected to die of it in 1993, when most of this book was written.

The prostate is a walnut-size gland located below the bladder and in front of the rectum. Surrounding the upper part of the urethra, the tube that carries urine from the bladder and semen from the prostate and the seminal vesicles, it needs male sex hormones to function. Testosterone, produced by the testicles, is the chief such hormone. Other male sex hormones are produced by the two adrenal glands, one gland being located above each kidney. Prostatic fluid is thick and comprises the major part of semen.

All cancer cells replicate too rapidly and behave in a disorderly fashion. They can spread to other parts of the body by means of the bloodstream and the lymphatic system. When prostate cancer spreads beyond the gland, it has a preference for lymph nodes and bones.

Although early detection and treatment have greatly increased, for unknown reasons the survival rate has not improved accordingly. It has been said prostate cancer is the most common malignancy in humans, but its cause is not understood. Treatment still often seriously injures sexual and/or urinary functions, and the prognosis for patients with advanced disease is disheartening. But there are bright, warm, brave, loving and humorous sides to this picture, as I believe the following narrative will show.

My hope is to offer readers the benefit not only of my experience but of the experience of others; to lead them step by step through what they are likely to encounter; and to help them understand and to cope.

Note

Where necessary, names have been changed to protect the privacy of persons and institutions.

I'm grateful to all the people who helped so generously in the making of this book.

One

Intermittent episodes of prostatitis (inflammation and/or infection of the prostate) over a period of fifteen to twenty years caused me continual apprehension about the possibility of my having prostate cancer, a concern that led to repeated examinations and batteries of tests. The tests included digital rectal exam, prostatic acid phosphatase, PSA (prostate-specific antigen), and transrectal ultrasound, none of which turned up anything alarming. Despite my relatively advanced age, I was in excellent physical condition, and my mental outlook, as I would occasionally be told by family and friends, was still youthful. I was feeling and working well, and was looking forward to an unspecified number of vigorous and on the whole useful and happy years.

And then came a routine, general physical exam early in 1993, my seventy-ninth year. After the exam, Dr. Daniel Redmont, my serious, formal and meticulous King City internist, said, "Your PSA is now 14.4, unusually high for you. I want the test repeated. Have blood drawn at the lab today."

The normal PSA range is 1 to 4. These numbers refer to nanograms (billionths of a gram of the antigen, a protein) per thousandth of a liter of blood. However, men with benign enlargement of the prostate may normally have a larger top number, as may men in their sixties and seventies. The currently very popular PSA test became widely available around 1987.

Dr. Redmont phoned me about a week later. "Your PSA is now 16.4," he said. "It's rising. I'm unhappy about it. Your prostate situation definitely needs to be reevaluated. I'm going to notify Dr. Lewis Gilroy [my King City urologist]. I urge you to see him promptly."

"What now?" I wondered. "Will this be just another false alarm? Or will it—finally—be the real thing? I'm symptom-free. So why the rise in my PSA? Ah, but cancer is stealthy. You can be feeling fine, while something deadly is happening inside you. What am I in for? God, I hope I don't have it."

"What's happening?" Joan, my wife, asked. "You look upset."

"I am."

I told her about Dr. Redmont's call and about my latest PSA, adding, "I've been too lucky. I have a feeling that this time I'm in for it," and immediately regretted having spoken so candidly. I was saddened by the look of anxiety that came over her and persisted throughout the evening.

"Are you sure PSA is reliable as a sign you have cancer?" she asked.

"The PSA indicates the rapidity with which prostate cells divide. And it does so with cancer cells as well as with benign ones. The cancer cells divide much more rapidly than the benign ones, which is why the PSA rises if you have cancer. Much depends on your PSA trend, and the trend in my case isn't good, it's upward. Daniel Redmont sounded almost a bit grim. And he was uncharacteristically silent about the digital exam he last gave me. I suspect he felt a tumor."

"Whatever happens, we'll deal with it," she said. "Remember, you're a survivor."

"Cancer is cancer. I doubt it respects survivors."

"Don't leap to conclusions."

"I'll try not to."

That evening I received two calls, one from Susy, my daughter, the other from Erik, my first-cousin.

"How's it going, Dad?" asked Susy.

When I briefly explained my prostate situation, I heard a change of tone in her voice. It's a cliché that the mere word, cancer, can create profound concern. I was sorry to share (and spread) anxiety, but Susy and I have always been open with each other concerning health matters.

Cousin Erik had a special interest in the possibility of my having prostate cancer, for he had been diagnosed with this cancer a little more than a year ago at the age of seventy-one, and had had a radical prostatectomy, resulting in a long period of incontinence and in permanent impotence. (Later, in an interview for the present narrative, Erik will describe his experience with his prostatectomy and its aftereffects.)

A radical prostatectomy involves surgical removal of the prostate, often accompanied by removal of the nearby lymph nodes. It can be accomplished, as in his case, by penetrating the abdomen, or by access through the perineal region, which in males is the area between the anus and the scrotum. I knew that the chance of one's getting prostate cancer is greater if one's father and/or brother has had it. True, Erik was a first cousin, not a brother, but I had a sense that his having had this cancer increased the possibility of my having it. Also, I knew that as one ages (and I am five years his senior), one is more likely to come down with it. We briefly discussed which course I should choose in the event I had it.

Being seventy-eight, I realized my time was short in any event. (You can argue with statistics just so far.) However, because I was in really good physical condition, with a brimming curiosity about many things in the world around me, my state of mind was not exactly that of a septuagenarian. Consequently I may have experienced a degree of anxiety more appropriate to a younger man.

FEBRUARY 12, 1993. This morning when I visited Dr. Gilroy, my urologist, who has an open, candid, friendly manner, with a

3

strong voice and a direct gaze, I had a long wait sitting alone on a gurney in a small room, getting overheated by a sterilizer and a bank of fluorescent ceiling lights, my trousers and undershorts down around my ankles. Dr. Gilroy entered, examined my genitals and gave my torso an extensive and thorough thumping.

"This hurt?" he asked during the pummeling. "I mean bone pain, not muscle pain. This hurt? This hurt?"

"No," I responded each time.

He was looking for symptoms of pain that might be due to prostate cancer. This form of cancer, if it breaks loose from the confines of the gland, tends to travel to bone, particularly in the pelvis and spine.

"Any pain in urinating? Any pain in the crotch?"

"No."

Though he said he'd be delicate, he gave me a prolonged and vigorous digital rectal exam, which the physician performs with a lubricated, latex-gloved finger. At moments I felt I had had enough; why was he continuing? As most men will probably agree, this is an embarrassing procedure at best. At times it can make you very uncomfortable. It can also make you feel you're about to urinate or ejaculate. At worst it can cause intense inner pain, especially if the physician, wishing to obtain a semen sample for microscopic analysis, massages the gland during a bout of prostatitis.

After getting dressed I went to his office. Saying there may be a suspicious protuberance in my prostate's left lobe, he prescribed a transrectal [via the rectum] ultrasound test, to be done in his office on the morning of February 25. In such an exam, sound waves inaudible to humans are emitted by a rectal probe. They bounce off the prostate, and a computer transforms the echoes into a picture called a sonogram.

"You have a very large gland," he said. "But I'm not worried about that. What worries me is that you have an elevated and increasing PSA. That, together with the suspicious spot, indicates we need to examine your gland with the ultrasound.

The three chief current modalities for detecting prostate cancer are a digital exam, the PSA, and the ultrasound. Prostate cancer and deaths due to it have been on the rise the past decade and no one is sure why. And the incidence increases with advancing age. You can't play God with a digital. Nor with the prostatic acid phosphatase and the prostate-specific antigen tests. Neither of them is sufficiently reliable for screening purposes. Today ultrasound is the state of the art. It's for men what mammography is for women. And it's approximately where mammography was some five or six years ago. In half a dozen years it'll be common. At present the chief resistance to it comes from insurance companies because of the expense. If you *have* cancer, Charley, we'll cure it."

An ultrasound exam gives good pictures of the prostate and is noninvasive, but it's expensive: $265. I'm to take no aspirin for at least a week before the test, in case he decides to do a biopsy. Aspirin encourages bleeding. Also, I'm to take a Fleet enema before coming to his office, and an antibiotic as a prophylactic measure. Before the development of the transrectal ultrasound, what you had was a random needle biopsy, mostly hit or miss. Using the ultrasound machine, the physician can see what he's doing.

I came away wondering what made Dr. Gilroy so sure he could cure my cancer if I had it. I told Joan what he had said. She was pleased and reassured. I also wondered why I had to wait until the 25th, thirteen days, for the ultrasound. Inasmuch as Dr. Gilroy apparently wasn't in a rush in my case, did it mean he wasn't seriously worried about the protuberance? I was ambivalent. On the one hand I was eager to have the ultrasound over with. On the other I was glad for the respite. Meanwhile I found myself thinking at times of what had happened to poor cousin Erik, and wondering if a similar fate was lurking for me.

There was snow to shovel in the driveway and slush to clear off the porch, and there were other house chores as well, and a

5

novella I was sketching, and President Bill Clinton's admirable address to a joint session of Congress, and *Unforgiven*, Clint Eastwood's powerful western. And, luckily for me, I was preoccupied (and on a high) with a class I was taking every Saturday morning at Mercer County Community College, some eight miles from my house, where I was learning how to make Cibachrome prints from some of my many Antarctic slides, a positive-to-positive system that requires working in complete darkness; and where I was also learning, unexpectedly, how strangely soothing, healing, the total darkness could be.

FEBRUARY 25. When I arrived at Dr. Gilroy's office for the ultrasound exam, a tall, friendly, middle-aged woman named Margaret, whom I hadn't met previously, led me to a restroom, where, alone, I removed my clothes below the waist and donned a blue gown open at the back. Then I went to the small ultrasound room, which contained a computer, a monitor and a black probe about the size of an erect penis. The probe was attached to the computer by a black electric cord. Fitting a condom on the probe, Margaret explained, "This is necessary to lessen the chance of spreading germs from one patient to another."

Dr. Gilroy, wearing a blue gown, entered, gave me a digital exam while Margaret was out of the room, and showed me how to lie on my left side, knees up toward my chest, on the gurney beside the machine. "I'm putting some xylocaine, a mild anaesthetic, on the probe," he said, and inserted the probe in my rectum. Margaret came in and turned out the lights. He moved the probe slowly and in various positions, occasionally saying, "I'd like a picture of that," after which I heard a click. In a while I stopped being embarrassed by Margaret's presence. But the procedure seeming lengthy, I began to be irritable. What was he seeing? What were *they* seeing? Why was he taking certain pictures and not others?

"What's he going to find?" I thought. "Do I have cancer? And if I do, is it curable? Will I live, but with a dreadfully changed quality of life? How will I handle bad news if it comes? It's extremely important to be graceful—graceful at all costs. And what about the protuberance? Why hasn't he mentioned it? Here I am, out in left field, and these two nice people, who are helping me, are healthy. Or at least they look healthy. But I look healthy too. What a confusion the human condition can be."

The pressure against parts of my prostate was increasingly unpleasant. When would he remove the damn probe? I wondered how long I could hold on. During the final part of the exam (measuring the gland) there were many fast clicks. He remarked to Margaret how very large my gland is.

"How you doing, Charley?" he asked.

"Fine," I replied in a strong, clear voice, surprising myself.

"I have to be careful and not miss anything," he said. "I work in a small town, and if I make a mistake I could be put out of business."

While I was still on my right side, knees flexed, he suddenly said, "I'm going to do a biopsy."

In a needle biopsy a fine, spring-powered needle is inserted into the rectum. Penetrating the rectal wall, the needle obtains prostate samples that are later examined by a pathologist. I felt something enter my rectum. I froze, expecting the procedure to be painful.

"Now there's going to be a bang," he warned.

The bang was loud, jolting me. I felt a nasty sting as the needle lunged into the gland, grabbed a specimen, and removed it. He repeated the procedure several times, occasionally asking Margaret, "Is the specimen okay?" Each time, she turned on the overhead lights and said, "It's fine," then doused them. The tension caused by the little crowded room, by the unfamiliar machine, by Margaret's presence (a strange woman *witnessing* the probe going into my rectum), by the procedure new to me, and above all by the suspense as to whether I have or don't have cancer, was badly tiring me and causing me to sweat.

Finally—at last!—he said, "That's it," and she turned the lights back on.

"How many specimens did you take?" I asked, my voice now soft and tentative.

"Seven. Five from the left lobe and two from the right. The right lobe looks good. The left looks uncertain. Get dressed, Charley, and wait for me in my office."

I returned to the restroom and wiped the gook off my bottom. In his office he showed me a long, narrow strip of black-and-white ultrasound photos of my prostate. Although I stared at them, I was unable to comprehend them; I was having trouble concentrating, and besides, they were weird looking.

"Because of its size, your gland produces more antigen than what we usually consider normal," Dr. Gilroy said. "We like to see the PSA reading under 8. Sometimes it runs to 12. In your case the size of the gland is at least partly responsible for the elevated number. We'll now have to wait for the pathology report. If you have cancer, much depends on two things: whether it has spread beyond the prostate, and the nature of the cell, whether it's mild, medium or aggressive. Call Helen [his office manager] tomorrow at 4:00 for the results."

In the evening, Cousin Erik, who has a well-developed sense of humor, called to hear my news, and gave me a great belly laugh by drily saying he was the self-proclaimed "President of the Limp Penis Club," a remark that a couple of hours later made me wonder, with a fair amount of anxiety, if I would soon become a charter member.

I'm not in the habit of praying, so when I went to bed that night I didn't pray to God to spare me from having prostate cancer. Once, more than two decades ago, I was involved in a near-fatal helicopter crash near the crest of Mount Erebus, a great active volcano in Antarctica. Three companions and I lay for many hours in a tiny Air Force survival tent before being rescued. Afterwards, when people asked me if I prayed for help, my response was, "No. Because I felt that the God who had put me there knew what He was doing, and wouldn't pay attention to my request for Him to change His mind."

As far as I know, Joan, my wife, didn't pray for me either, but I noticed how extremely supportive of me she was being because of the possibility I had cancer. I'm by no means suggesting that prayer isn't a great good thing. I probably have my own way of praying, which is not readily recognizable to me as part of that rubric.

FEBRUARY 26, 1993, FRIDAY. I tried to work on my novella as if this was an ordinary day, but I was too distracted by suspense and my awareness of time as I waited to call Helen in Dr. Gilroy's office at 4:00 for the pathologist's report.

"Let's get it over with," I kept thinking.

If the biopsy was negative, what a relief that would be! Still, at seventy-eight such relief is a joke, in a way, because, as the man wrote in *Hamlet*, "If it be not now, yet it will come. The readiness is all." If it was positive. . . . If it was positive, even at best my life would undergo profound and hard-to-predict changes.

I struggled, much of the day, to be optimistic. It didn't help to learn, in a call from Cousin Erik, that my first cousin Murray, who had some months ago completed a course of radiation for prostate cancer, was now probably impotent. Radiation can damage the two erectile nerves, one on either side of the prostate, that are involved in penile erection. It does this not necessarily by hurting the nerves directly, but often by adversely affecting capillaries and tissues that nourish the nerves. How did Erik know this about Murray? Well, yesterday Murray had called Erik to ask about the vacuum method for achieving an erection, something Erik had investigated, trying it out after buying the equipment and its attendant videotape illustrating its use. [Erik will describe his experience with the method later in this narrative.]

When at last it was 4:00 I felt free to call Helen. A woman I didn't know said Helen wasn't in. "Just my luck. Just when I need her, she isn't in," I thought, as if Helen, whom I had always found to be unusually friendly and responsible, had signed a contract with me to be in place for my call.

When I explained the purpose of my call, the woman promptly said, "The girl hasn't come yet with the results. I'll call you one way or the other before leaving the office."

She wasn't as good as her word, and I soon found myself increasingly suspenseful and irritable. What *would* the pathologist's report say? By now, I almost desperately had to know. I needed to know where I stood. Anything to stop the painful suspense. Not hearing from a soul by 4:30, I phoned Dr. Gilroy's home in King City and asked his wife to have him call me. He returned the call around 6:30.

"What's the news?" I asked.

"It's not good."

"I have cancer?"

"Yes. In the left lobe."

"So now, at last, I *know*," I thought, and my ground-floor study, surrounded on three sides by a yard and trees, in which I had taken his call, seemed to darken. "Everything has changed. From now on cancer isn't *out there*. It's the enemy *inside me*, eating away at something vital." I experienced the cliché sinking feeling, as if something had suddenly happened to my blood pressure.

The type of cancer cell, as far as I could understand him (this was before I knew about the all-important Gleason score), was 3 plus 3; or 6, meaning midway between mild and aggressive.

"It's not too bad," he said, trying to reassure me. "If you had a 9 or a 10 . . . you could start thinking of a pine box."

Pretty blunt talk. Even shocking talk, it seemed to me. It had the flavor of a Western film. I wondered if he had seen a Western recently. I saw myself stretched out in a pine box. Still juiced up and irritable from the day's suspense, and probably angry because I had cancer, I felt myself ready to be judgmental about him.

"The first two areas a prostate cancer is likely to reach after leaving the gland are bone and lymph nodes," he explained. "On Monday, Helen will set up appointments for you to have a bone scan and a CAT scan at the hospital. After we get the results of these tests, we'll meet to discuss what steps we should take."

"Lew, we've taken care," I said. "We've watched the situation closely. How did it manage to get out of hand?"

"Charley, I don't know the answer to that," he replied, a bit testily. "If I did, I'd be a genius."

Was he being overworked? Was he irritated because I had called his home? But he had offered no explanation as to why my call to his office had been fruitless. And this was my life we were dealing with. Or maybe my death?

I had a hunch my cancer had traveled. In Erik's case there had been a discreet lump; in Cousin Murray's there had been two lumps. These facts suggested for me that their prostate cancer had been localized. In my case, as I understood it, there was no lump. (I was jumping the gun, and being irrational, and unnecessarily pessimistic. What was the suspicious protuberance if not a lump?) My cancer struck me as being amorphous; that is, that it wasn't encapsulated. And for this reason, I believed, it was more likely to have traveled outside the gland. I was accepting, on very dubious evidence, a worst-case scenario for myself. Why, I don't know. Did my state of mind have to do with my advanced age, and consequently a more ready acceptance of death—or rather, not of actual death, with all the vivid facts of physical dissolution, but of the idea, an abstraction, of my mortality? Do some people take an equally irrational optimistic view?

On the other hand, there was a real possibility my cancer had traveled (the fancy word is metastasized). Otherwise, why did I need bone and CAT scans? I thought back to the time, some four years earlier, when a New York urologist had wanted to do a random biopsy on me, one without an ultrasound. I had declined. I wondered now if he had been right in suspecting I had cancer. Maybe I had had the cancer even then, and that it had flourished for four long years, with the possibility of spreading.

"I'm just sorry for *you*, having to deal with the crap that's coming," I said to Joan in the kitchen.

"I'm determined to be optimistic about you," she responded. "Remember, you're a survivor."

It was the kind of reaction I expected from her. Born in Vancouver, she had been raised in Concord, Massachusetts, and educated at Concord Academy, Vassar and Columbia University. (She had been awarded a doctorate in German literature by Columbia.) She has a wonderfully stoical, New England streak. We had known each other a long time. In August 1952 I was writing a book at the Huntington Hartford Foundation, an artists' colony in Rustic Canyon in Pacific Palisades, California, and occasionally meeting with my friend Thomas Mann, the great German novelist, who lived in Pacific Palisades then. She came from Vienna at the conclusion of a Fulbright in German literature, and we got married in Santa Monica that month. She had been marvelously supportive all those years, and had never made me feel in the least guilty for going off to Antarctica on three occasions, on one of them almost failing to come back.

Despite the bad news, we had a pleasant dinner, during which I told myself to try to stop thinking about such questions as "Will I be able to attend the Antarctic workshop [sponsored by the Office of Polar Programs of the National Science Foundation] in Boulder in May?" and "Will I be able to housesit, as promised, for my friends Peter and Penny Kenez in Aptos, California in July?"

FEBRUARY 27, SATURDAY. My Cibachrome printing class ran from 9:00 to 2:00 each Saturday. I looked forward to the sessions and was sorry when they ended, even if I was very tired.

I decided to keep my cancer from the class, not because I was secretive or because I was ashamed of it, but because I needed a respite from it, needed to avoid thinking about it all the time, and because I believed it would be unfair to lay that knowledge on my classmates, all of whom were a great deal younger than I and who hadn't taken the class in order to deal with heavy medical news.

Two youngish female classmates seemed to enjoy chatting with me, consequently my secret knowledge made me unusually shy, especially when I wondered if I would soon join the Limp Penis Club. In addition, no doubt because of my age, I was aware that I was beginning to view human sexual activities from a great distance, and to wonder what all the sexual fuss was about (violent jealousy; rape; murder; the Othello complex; Tolstoy's *The Kreutzer Sonata* came to mind). Also, I recalled the human awareness, at certain stages, of life's limitations, and I thought that Annie Donnelly, my granddaughter (the daughter of Susy and Whitney, my son-in-law), not yet four, so vibrant with beauty and life, if she was lucky would reach old age, with some or many of its infirmities.

Mostly I was able to keep my mind on my Cibachrome work, but at certain moments today in the completely dark, small processor room in which I locked myself to prevent an accidental opening of the door and a consequent breach of the darkness, I felt the need to cry. I had a deep, painful sense of mourning, as if I had just lost a person dear to me. "The person you're mourning is yourself," I thought. "Pull yourself together. Whatever happens will happen. Remember Mount Erebus. You've already died, in a way. That fact should steady you, whatever's in store."

Emotionally it was an unsteady time for me. Sometimes, alone at home, handling a knife, I had a fleeting wish to cut myself; at others to swallow a handful of sleeping pills. But I thought of how much trouble it would cause Joan and Susy, and how let down, how scarred, certain friends would be. Joan

13

would possibly understand. She had sometimes heard me say, echoing Borges, the Argentine writer, "I'm tired of being Neider. I've been around too long. There's too long a stretch between Bessarabia and World War I and now." (I was born in Odessa and spent some childhood years in Akkerman, a town in Bessarabia on the western shore of the Dniester estuary. Since 1940 Akkerman has been called Belgorod-Dniestrovski.)

There was an accident in the processor room today while I was alone in it. My 8×10 paper, sliding face down, had not quite disappeared into the machine's bowels, and I was closing the processor door, when some metal trays with pointed ends cascaded with a loud clatter onto me from a high shelf, striking my right cheek and the right side of my nose. Some fell into the still open door. I removed two trays from the processor door, felt for my paper, felt the end of it disappearing, closed the door, closed my paper safe, and carrying the latter, left the room and reentered the brilliantly illuminated central workroom, where a couple of women, classmates, glanced sharply at me.

"You're bleeding," remarked one. Touching my nose and seeing blood on my finger, I realized I was lucky not to have been hit in the eye.

"What happened?" asked somebody. I explained.

"Go to the men's room and apply a cold wet paper towel," said Kay Hymans, the assistant teacher, looking and sounding unusually serious. In class she often wore an ironic smile, though she was an altogether pleasant person. "I mean it! Do it *now!*" I promptly went there and did as I was told. Worried looks from Lou Draper, the teacher, who had followed me into the men's room to ask if I was ok.

"I'm fine," I said.

When I returned to the workroom, Kay, saying I was still bleeding, applied paper towels to my face and asked me to hold them there until the bleeding stopped.

Laughing, I said, "Shame on you! You're not wearing latex gloves! Suppose I have AIDS?"

"Oh, you!" she cried. Trying to sound stern while laughing, she said, "Now don't you dare laugh! When you laugh, your nose starts bleeding again!"

"If you only knew my secret," I thought. "I have cancer, and by comparison with that, I wouldn't care much if the accident had removed the tip of my nose."

When my print emerged from the chemical processor and I put it face up into a bath of agitated water, Sylvia, a pretty woman, one of the two classmates I've already mentioned, noticed that an end had a blip where it had been struck by a point that had almost pierced the paper, which, though it was called paper, was heavy, untearable polyester. Again I realized how lucky I had been not to be hit in the eye. My luck was by no means all bad, I thought.

That evening, at a moment when I was tired and depressed, Susy called and said, "Annie's whining. She wants to talk to you. Is it okay?"

"Sure. How are you?" I asked Annie.

"Good!"

"Did you have a nice day?"

"Yes!"

"Great. Now I need to speak with your mommy. Your mommy wants to speak with me."

"It's not going to be like that today," said this person crisply who wasn't yet four; who was almost three-quarters of a century my junior.

I cracked up. She was right to object to my trying to dump her like that. I was right too, because she had a habit of hanging onto the phone (and me) as if time was an inexpressibly cheap commodity, as indeed it was, for *her*. Anyhow, we kept chatting, until Susy, sensing my predicament, rescued me by taking the phone away from her. There was no way I could rescue myself from this granddaughter of mine. And yet I believed, as I was willing to tell anyone who would listen, that I didn't have the normal grandparent's extreme admiration of a grandchild; that my love of Annie was mostly aesthetic, due to her charm and beauty.

Often, when I was feeling down, I yearned to see Annie, to enjoy her brightness, beauty, gentleness, social intelligence, love of laughter—and female coyness. Despite the cancer I now had to deal with, on the whole my own vigor, my own involvement with life, my own laughter seemed as rich as ever.

Two

March 4 to March 10, 1993

MARCH 4, 1993. I arrived at the King City Medical Center at 9:15 A.M., checked in, and was told to have a seat in the nuclear medicine section. A young brunette nurse soon called me, said, "I'm Carolyn. Come with me," and led me with a smile to a small room. She was carrying what looked like a heavy green thermos, out of the top of which stuck a syringe plunger. I sat down and rolled up my sleeve. She found a vein. Turning my head away, I felt a tiny sting.

"What's this for?" I asked.

"I've injected a radioactive material. It will attach itself only to the calcium and phosphorus in your bones," she explained. "It will emit gamma rays. Try to avoid children and pregnant women for twenty-four hours."

"I was looking forward to hugging my little granddaughter today."

"Just don't get close to her."

"Am I through now?"

"Here? Yes."

As I approached the nuclear medicine waiting area on my way out of the hospital, I noticed a seated young woman in a green hospital gown. She had light brown hair, was attached to an IV, and was crying, and dabbing at her eyes with a paper tissue while an older woman, a squatting nurse in white, was trying to comfort her. "Poor lady. God knows what's in store for her," I thought.

I was home by 10:00 and back at the hospital by 12:30. I checked in at the Radiology Department and sat down in the waiting room. A tall, stately young woman in white, with very blue eyes, carrying three astonishingly large white styrofoam cups on a white styrofoam tray, approached me.

"Are you Mr. Neider?" she asked, looking down at me.

"Yes."

She handed me the tray. One cup had scrawled on it in black ink, *NOW*; a second, *1:15*; the third, *2:00*. "Drink the first now," she instructed. "It's for your CAT scan."

"I'm having a bone scan at 1:00."

"Oh. Follow me."

She led me to the nuclear medicine waiting area. "The restroom's down the hall. Good idea to use it," she said. "Drink the second cup during a bone scan break." She left.

"Cocktails before lunch," I remarked to a large, stout woman sitting on my left, lifting the cup as if for a toast, and reaching for a copy of *Newsweek* on a chair. The woman smiled but said nothing. A heavyset man in a brown suit, joining her, spoke to her in Russian.

Again I was astonished by the size of the cups. (Later I learned that each contained about 16 ounces of a liquid whose function was to highlight my stomach, intestines and colon.) Using the straw, I began drinking. An effort had been made to suggest lemonade in this concoction, but the taste brought visions of gagging. Having been instructed to have only a liquid lunch today, I had filled myself with chicken broth. So I wasn't surprised when, immediately on finishing the cup, I urgently had to pee. I went to the restroom down the corridor. It was composed of two rooms. The first was a cluttered anteroom: bedpans, chairs, gauze, latex examination gloves, syringes. I locked myself in, relieved myself, washed and dried my hands, returned to my seat, and soon was summoned for my bone scan by a brown-skinned, reserved woman whom I followed to a small, dimly lit room crowded with equipment.

"Empty your trousers of any metal, please," she said. "And remove your belt buckle and glasses."

"What about my wristwatch?"

"You can keep that on."

With my shoes on, I lay down on a table barely wider than my waist. It was covered by a strip of green foam mattress containing conical little hills.

"Why is this table so narrow?" I asked.

"It's so the gamma camera can get close to you. The closer it is, the greater the resolution. The camera will photograph your gamma rays."

She handed me a broad, strong, elliptical, dark-colored ribbon, and showed me how to thrust my arms through it. Arranging the ribbon across the lower part of my chest, I grasped its function: to support my arms at my sides.

"Lie extremely still," she said, arranging a tight elastic band around my feet.

The upper lights went out, leaving a deep twilight. The camera, a thick, round, large, white machine that approached various parts of my body, at times almost touched my face. "Joan wouldn't like this at all," I thought. She had startled me many years ago in the Carlsbad Caverns when we were in a vast room, with a mighty ceiling. Suddenly, looking pale and shaky, she had said, "Please take me out of here. I'm not getting enough oxygen." It was my first realization she's susceptible to claustrophobia. I, on the other hand, have never experienced it, even during submarine diving exercises in the North Atlantic, or in the close bowels of a heaving icebreaker on the Southern Ocean. We had headed promptly for an elevator that took us to the surface. Now, in the bone scan room, I became aware of machine-made clicks. After a while I fell asleep.

"Turn your head to the right," said the brown-skinned, formal lady technician.

Opening my eyes, I was surprised to see a bright computer screen with a death's head on it, brilliant in blue and white. I gathered these were the bones of my head (skull, teeth, jaws) in a picture created by my radioactive emissions, the gamma camera and a computer. Then I saw another view, a frontal one of my head and chest. Did those ruby reds on places I took to be my esophagus, or stomach, or lungs indicate the presence of cancer cells? Closing my eyes, I thought, "No time to be the Great Diagnostician. Don't listen to him, heart."

I was in the bone scan room about an hour, except for a brief intermission, during which I urgently visited the restroom, then drank the cup marked *1:15*. I returned to the waiting room, drank the third cup of liquid, and traipsed to the restroom six or seven times. It became increasingly hard for me to start and stop peeing.

Occasionally I noticed some new patient in the crowded corridor, brought there by elevator, and almost invisible under covers on a gurney. A man of about forty, with reddish eyes, a reddish mustache, a stubble beard and a roguish look, was sitting hunched over in a wheelchair, his naked back exposed by the opening in his green hospital gown. Our eyes met. I was unable to read the message in his. I gave him a friendly look. An elderly man, propped in a sitting position, stared with bulging, unseeing gray eyes. Was he comatose? Drugged?

A woman summoned me for the CAT scan. I followed her into the CAT scan room. Another woman said in a tone that suggested she was giving me a hug, "Hello, honey, how are you? I'm Christina. Lie on the table. I'm going to put a sheet over your waist. When I do, unzip your trousers and pull them down to your knees. We don't want the zipper to be in the way."

She left the room. A younger nurse entered and attached an IV, by which I received a liquid that, she explained, would highlight certain of my blood vessels. "The CAT scan uses X rays. So I'm going to leave the room to avoid them," she said.

"Stop breathing," soon came her command in a hollow, loud, metallic sound over a speaker. I took a breath and held it. *"Breathe."* And so on.

Obvious thoughts kept crowding my mind. Such as, "These tests will determine a great deal—my fate." Or, "It's necessary to do all this to get a handle on my condition—to know whether the damn cancer has escaped the gland. And if so, to what extent." Irritated by them, I tried to shove them out of my head. But they wouldn't leave; or if they did, it was only for a pathetically little while. They made me feel like an idiot. For what was the point of repeating such obvious thoughts? In addition, I felt I was being judged in some way. But what was my crime? "Old age," a stern, prosecutor's voice in me said. "The older a man is, the more likely he'll get prostate cancer. That's the *law* in these parts." At one point I had a feeling that was more appropriate to enacting a scene in *High Noon*.

There's nothing like a battery of hospital tests to make you feel vulnerable, naked; as if your very life depends on them. As, indeed, it may. I had been living a quiet life, minding my business, not breaking the law. My time had felt free; which was what I had been used to; which I had always wanted; and still wanted. And now, suddenly, I was caught up in the full-fledged machinery of cancer; the machinery of what felt like a WAR. Tests. Questions. Debates. Crucial decisions. What was the enemy's local strength, position, logistics, tactics? What was his strategy? Above all, who would win?

When my CAT scan was finished, I peed again before heading for home. By the time I reached my garaged car I needed to go again. I had to go urgently at home fifteen minutes later. It took three or four hours for my bladder to calm down.

"What now?" I wondered when I turned in. "Will I learn the answer tomorrow? And if I do, what will it be?"

MARCH 5, 1993, 11:15 A.M. I have a 3:45 appointment with Dr. Gilroy today, at which time I'm to learn if my cancer has left the prostate and entered the nearby lymph nodes and bones. If it has, I have two choices: I can ignore the situation, or I can accept therapy. Therapy might mean hormone treatment (medical castration); or surgical castration; and possibly also radiation. On the other hand, if the cancer is contained, I can watchfully wait; or have surgery or radiation. I've seen the consequences of a radical prostatectomy on Cousin Erik: pain; a long period of incontinence; a long recovery time; probably permanent impotence.

Cousin Murray, who had had a TURP (a transurethral resection of the prostate, an operation that reams out and removes some of the tissues of an enlarged gland), with a long recovery time and some incontinence, chose radiation. He and his wife, Jan, return from Florida at the end of the month. He'll get a PSA soon thereafter. It will be interesting to learn from it what the radiation did for him.

Calling me this morning, Erik said he's hoping for the best in my case. "Thanks. But I'm seventy-eight," I said wryly. "How much longer can I expect to stay in good health?" Erik's doctor, Fledermaus, told him radiation is a palliative, that only a radical prostatectomy is a cure, and that there's only one kind of cell in prostate cancer. Bullshit. I've read enough to know that radiation is a great deal more than a "palliative," and that the cells range from timid to aggressive. Fledermaus is a knife-man; he preaches what he practices; prostatectomy is his thing; but why does he have to lie about the cancer cells?

2:15 P.M. I just returned from lunch with Bernie Breitbart and found a message that Dr. Gilroy wants to see me at 2:45, an hour earlier than scheduled. Lunch at Forrestal Village, near Princeton, was very pleasant. It was only when I received Dr. Gilroy's message that my cancer problem returned to my mind and emotions. It's all so relative. Now it would be great news to learn my cancer hasn't spread a good deal, or spread at all. I told Joan I'm not optimistic. I begin to see the value of religion, whose chief gift, it seems, is the belief we'll all meet in a hereafter.

I drive to the Medical Center garage but find no parking spot except on the roof, where it's snowing, slushy and slippery. "Don't complicate matters with a bad fall," I tell myself as I walk carefully to Dr. Gilroy's office. Dr. Gilroy is with an emergency patient. Alone in the waiting room, I hear his voice behind a closed door. I leave the sofa to stare out the window at the street, where large snowflakes are gently falling.

What's in store for me? Good news? Bad? *Very* bad? Has my cancer spread to bones, and am I in for some bad pain? Is my lifestyle about to undergo a change (not to mention my quality of life)? A truck lumbers down the street as if nothing unusual is happening. What have my scans shown? What does Dr. Gilroy *know* that he'll have to share with me any moment now? How many times has he given men very bad news? And how have they taken it?

After about forty-five minutes, Gilroy strides into the waiting room with a hearty "Hi Charley!" and a strong handshake. Clearly, the world's all fine with him today, or he's putting up a good front. I follow him into his office. "Now, let's take a look at where you stand," he says, picking up a large reddish envelope on his desk. "The bone scan first." He shoves a series of pictures onto the light wall on my right. Speaking as if to himself, he checks each bone carefully. "This is okay. This is okay. Here's your femur. This is your skull, Charley."

Standing on his right and slightly behind him, I wonder if he has already read the pathologist's report. Does he already know what the verdict is? Strange . . . you move along . . . you do your life . . . all seems well, relatively serene . . . and meanwhile your fate has hit slippery ground . . . and you're not aware of it . . . until now, when judgment is about to be handed down by a sort of court clerk.

"Well, *that's* all clear," he says. "Now let's look at the CAT scan."

He slips the CAT scan pictures vigorously under the hidden springs on the wall. There are many pictures. "If the cancer

23

doesn't kill you, the radiation or prostatectomy may," I think. "But for an old cocker like me it hardly matters." He goes over the pictures carefully, checking out organs while speaking softly to himself. "The left kidney looks okay in this shot. Okay in this shot. Okay here too. Left kidney's clear. Let's take a look at the right one." Occasionally he interrupts himself to speak directly to me, but without turning to face me. "A little lesion in your chest cavity. Some arthritis in the right shoulder. This is your heart. You have a large aorta. What a huge prostate! Look at that! Isn't it large?"

For Christ's sake! I think. Why is he handing me all these details? Who cares about the details? They're means to an end, not an end in themselves! All I want to know is—has my cancer spread? And if so, how far? Give me the verdict first, and *then* the details. And if the verdict is good, I'll *enjoy* the details. If he hasn't already read the pathologist's report, why not? It was his job to do it, and not to study the pictures for the first time while in my presence! Doesn't he realize the suspense I'm in, and that this dillydallying with details is cruel? Give it to me now is what I want! Quit stalling! Was he too busy to read the report? But if he's overscheduled, is that *my* problem? If *he* had prostate cancer, would *he* want to be treated like this?

It takes about a half-hour for him to check all the images. Finally he says, "Well, in my judgment this is not an incurable situation. Everything's clear."

He puts the pictures away and sits down at his desk. Sitting down too, facing him, I feel my suspenseful, angry body beginning to relax.

"Of course, if I had a cross-section of the lymph nodes under a microscope, I might find cancer cells," he continues. "I don't know. Nobody knows—without operating on you. But as far as these pictures are concerned, everything's clear."

"That's good enough for me," I say. "Lew, I'm surprised."

"Why?"

"I was wrong. I expected the cancer to have traveled."

"Why?"

"Because it seemed amorphous."

"Well, Charley, it hasn't."

Dr. Gilroy outlines my options. One: I can ignore the cancer. Two: I can opt for a prostatectomy. And three: I can go for radiation.

"I'm not going to tell you what to do," he says. "It's not my way. However, let me tell you this. Studies have shown that surgery and X-ray therapy are equal modalities for a ten-year survival rate. For a fifteen-year survival rate, surgery moves ahead a bit."

I planned to make a decision jointly with Joan, but now I have no hesitation in deciding unilaterally. To repeat, I've seen what a radical prostatectomy did to Erik. On the other hand, maybe Erik had a more aggressive cancer cell than I. He doesn't know the type he had. By lying to him, his urologist deprived him of the opportunity to make an extremely important decision regarding himself. If I have surgery, I'll be inactive for a long time. I'm in good shape for seventy-eight and want to stay that way a while longer. I don't know what side effects I'll have with radiation but I'm optimistic, I feel I'll be able to continue my power walks, travels and work.

"What I see is a healthy man," Dr. Redmont, my internist, said after my annual physical. A healthy man with cancer.

"What are we talking about? I'm seventy-eight. Ten years is a long time at my age. I'll go for radiation," I tell Dr. Gilroy.

"If I were you, Charley, that's what I'd do."

"I need to be in Boulder for an Antarctic workshop May 7 to 9."

"No problem."

"And in California for July."

"No problem there either."

As I rise from my chair he hands me a printed sheet. "What's this?" I ask.

"The pathology report on the biopsy."

"I'm surprised, Lew," I repeat as we're leaving his office.

25

He glances at me quizzically. "You're happy, aren't you?" he asks.

"Sure, but I'll be damned if I beg for life."

In the corridor I clap him fondly on his strong back. He asks Helen to set up an appointment with a radiation oncologist at the Medical Center. The first doctor she tries won't be back until March 30. I say I don't want to wait that long, so she makes an appointment with another, Edward North, for the 11th. As it turns out, it's by such a small accident that I select the perfect oncologist for myself.

Heading for the garage, feeling confused, stepping carefully in the slush, I realize I need to adjust my thinking to a more optimistic mode. The cancer hasn't spread! I won't need hormone therapy! Glancing at the hospital entrance, I vividly recall the unhappy scenes in the nuclear medicine section I witnessed yesterday. With these in mind, it's impossible for me to jump up and down inwardly like a child because I've been "spared." Still, in the garage I sense I'm smiling. "What a nice car you are," I think as I slip into it.

The streets feel unusually friendly. I park in my garage more gently than usual. Joan is upstairs. Hearing me enter, she comes down.

"Well?" she asks, trying to read my eyes.

"All clear."

She pummels me with her fists. "I was right!" she cries, glowing with relief and pleasure. "I was right to be optimistic! I told you you're a survivor!"

There are calls to be made, people's nerves to be spared. Swallowing a handsome amount of Absolut, I proceed to make them. Later I'll learn that Kate Doyle, an old and dear friend, prayed for me and asked other people to pray. And that Susy, my daughter, wore a special good-luck charm during several crucial days. I didn't pray. It seemed distasteful to ask God for a special favor. I had already been granted a great favor in being healthy, vigorous and free for so long.

It's very pleasant, of course, conveying good news, and receiving calls of congratulation. My brother, Mark, and his wife, Mildred, call and say they'll drive to Princeton tomorrow from Dobbs Ferry, New York, where they live, and celebrate my news with a dinner out that will include Susy, Whitney and Annie. My sister, Tessie Noble, and her husband, Sam, call from Floria. Not the least part of the fun I have in making these calls stems from the fact that I genuinely expected metastasis, and am still very surprised by the good news brought by the scans.

I call my friend Tom Hunter in Keswick, Virginia, a remarkable man who got polio at the age of seven, yet had a wonderful career in medicine. I think, "Tom lives with congestive heart failure, yet he still goes to his office in Charlottesville, still does grand rounds, is still keenly interested in the larger world.

Once, speaking recently to me about his polio, he said, "I got it in 1920, the same year as Franklin Roosevelt. But I wasn't 'struck down.' It was the greatest thing that could have happened to me. It saved my life. Without it I would have become a businessman. I've had a great life, Charles. The only reason I stay alive, Charles, is I do so little. Any little exertion tires me badly." He reassures me now. "Even if the cancer had spread," he says, "you'd probably have ten good years ahead of you. Modern medicine is doing remarkable things in preserving human life."

"Tom, I've been a free man all my life. And now I think I'm no longer free."

"You son of a bitch," he says, "don't you dare whine about losing your freedom. You've had one of the freest lives I know."

"I love you, Tom. Do you know that?"

"I think I do," he says, now softly, distantly.

Emotionally almost exhausted, I turned in early that evening, but before doing so I read the biopsy report, which confirmed I have adenocarcinoma (cancer) confined to the left lobe, with a Gleason score of 6. Dr. Gilroy hadn't mentioned my Gleason

27

number; or, for that matter, Gleason numbers in general. Why not? (I learned later that Gleason numbers [or scores] are very important, because they can be accurately predictive regarding the outcome of prostate cancer.) And why hadn't Dr. Fledermaus, Erik's urologist, informed *him* about Gleason numbers, and told him his number? And Cousin Murray's urologist, too, hadn't mentioned Gleason scores to Murray, or offered to give him *his* score. However, Murray had told me he wasn't interested in such details; that the less he knew about the details of his condition (including the details of radiation therapy), the happier he was. My view is different from Murray's. I want to know as much as possible, for intellectual reasons; but also, and primarily, because I want to participate in making decisions that can affect my health and possibly my survival. I resent being kept in the dark by doctors. I dislike playing the trusting, blind child with them, because I know from experience that, like all humans, they're fallible.

I'm belaboring this point in the hope of convincing readers to take a direct and personal interest in their cancer. My cousin Erik, as I believe we'll see during the progress of this narrative, suffered—how grievously, he can best say—from a lack of information his urologist ought to have supplied him. The problem with us novices is that we don't know which questions to ask. We count on the doctors to provide us with the questions. Of course, I respect Murray's view, and maybe it works best for him. It would not be good for me.

Anyway, that evening I wondered why Dr. Gilroy had failed to communicate details of my biopsy report while spending so much time commenting about my bone and CAT scans. I'm genuinely fond of him. Clapping him on the back after our light-screen session wasn't hypocritical. But, in my opinion, his behavior during the session was faulty, and at my expense.

NEXT DAY, SATURDAY. I got up at 5:00 and was at the Cibachrome lab at 8:00. Working without a lunch break, I made five 8 × 10 glossy prints. I always worked with glossy paper rather than with matte; the glossy, though more expensive, was superior in color richness and in image resolution. I had a great deal of trouble with flecks of dirt, and with poor processor chemistry. Classroom work has its obvious limitations when measured against a privately owned lab. Lab cleanliness in the class was beyond my control, as was the freshness of the chemistry and the condition of the processor. Still, I was happy to take the class, and I sympathized with my two teachers, who also lacked the necessary control.

Frustrated and irritated, I got home at 3:30 and found that Mark and Mildred and Susy and Susy's family were waiting for me. The celebration dinner, with wine, was excellent, with much laughter, and my mood soon improved. Annie, age four, behaved beautifully. For me, the only sour note occurred in the restaurant in the form of a large solitary fish that looked depressed as it swam listlessly in a too-small tank.

Several days later, studying the radiologists' report on my bone and CAT scans (a copy of which I had obtained from Dr. Gilroy's office), I learned that the gamma camera had obtained views of my skull, spine, ribs, sternum, pelvis and hips; and that the bone scan was normal; that is, it found no evidence of increased bone activity. (The isotope, a radioactive material, that was injected into me is attracted to bone cells that are replicating with unusual speed, which is what cancer cells do.) Also, the CAT scan, made of my abdomen and pelvis, had checked my lungs, liver, spleen, adrenal glands, pancreas and kidneys. The radiologists found all to be normal; my seminal vesicles were normal in size and were symmetric. My prostate was markedly enlarged.

I thought, "So here's the verdict. It's easy enough to read it quickly. Had Dr. Gilroy read it? If so, why did he put on the light-screen show that kept me in such painful suspense? Was he being friendly, taking me into an inner sanctum? Or had he played the scene for its greatest dramatic effect?"

Whatever. . . . The result was a good verdict. . . . I was in the clear. . . . The cancer hadn't spread (so far as one knew without a microscopic examination of my lymph nodes). . . . Yes, I was in the clear . . . with prostate cancer. Here was the heart of the relativity of disease. It could be worse . . . much worse. . . . And, despite my advanced age, I was very happy it wasn't, and so were the people close to me who knew about my condition.

I went, one day, with my friend and neighbor, Bernie Breitbart, to Mercerville, Pennsylvania, to pick up some printed cocktail glasses for his Princeton sailing club. The shop was dingy and poorly lit. The cluttered front office was run by a tall older man wearing a very tired cap.

"You're lean. You look in great shape," I said.

"Think so?" he asked, brightening. "I used to weigh 298. Now I weigh 189."

"What happened?"

"My doc told me to knock it off or I'd better select a casket. So I started eating nothing but grapefruit."

"How old are you?"

"69."

"You don't look it."

"I had my prostate reamed. I'm doing okay. Except. You know Hawaiian? I'll talk Hawaiian to you. Lackanooky."

I responded with a belly laugh.

"You Irish?" I asked.

"That's me."

"My cousin Erik had his prostate out," I said. "He says, 'I'm the President of the Limp Penis Club.'"

A great burst of laughter from the man.

MARCH 10, 1993. Erik invited Joan and me to visit Molly and him this weekend. I declined because, thinking of driving to Irvington, it occurred to me that if I'm involved in a car accident, it may hold up my X-ray therapy, and that there's no way of knowing how long the cancer cells will wait patiently inside my gland until they're killed. Suppose they grow restless. Rebellious. Angry. I'd better stay on good terms with them. What if they have an inside track with the mysterious mechanism which, years ago, with self-hypnosis, eliminated without a trace the growth on my left eye's lower lid? Better not take them too much for granted, or be too readily comforted by the high tech of the computer-operated X rays that will soon start zapping me.

When I related to my friend John Lowrance at lunch today some of my bawdy cancer anecdotes, he smiled and laughed, but with restraint, almost with pain, like the good, proper Gentile he is. John, who took early retirement at Princeton University and heads a company he formed, Princeton Scientific Instruments, is developing, with FDA support, a machine that will test condoms with ultraviolet light.

More evidence that Cousin Murray has become impotent. He recently called Erik—again—to ask about the vacuum method of achieving an erection. Molly answered the phone.

"What's up, Murray?" she asked, unaware of the double entendre.

"I've joined the club," Murray confided to Erik. "The club of which you're president."

"Maybe his impotence is temporary," said Erik to me. "Maybe at ninety he'll be able to get it up."

We howled—not with any hostility to Murray, but over the wildness of the Human Kondition.

Three

March 11 to March 18, 1993

Before I knew the extent of my cancer, before I was secure in the knowledge it hadn't spread, I felt at times alone, with the sense that all of us are alone when it comes to dying, unless we have religion or some equivalent to bolster us. But I was ready to go, if need be. Only a young man could have written Dylan Thomas's "Rage, rage against the dying of the light." Raging in this context strikes me, at seventy-eight, as graceless. I admire Socrates, who drank his cup of hemlock with style, and Robert Falcon Scott, who died quietly and bravely in the tent on the vast Ross Ice Shelf in Antarctica.

I lived in a world of averages, probability. How did I know my cancer wasn't preparing to leave the gland next week to do some fancy traveling? What would happen if I had a car accident that would delay my X-ray therapy? Would my cancer be delighted because of its greater chance of survival?

One night I dreamed I was a colonel in the army, wearing khaki and getting a lot of respect. I particularly liked wearing khaki. I also dreamed I was cursorily examining a large-format book of pictures of Antarctica and deciding that the layout and photographs weren't all that good. I awoke feeling high. Joan asked if I had had a good sleep. I replied I had had a great one and told her about the dreams. I was full of laughter, which made her laugh too. I had taken a Temazepam sleeping pill that night. It was a fine drug that reduced my (age-caused?) aches and pains. At times I thought that if I could take it for six months without side effects, it might free me of them. A recent article in the *New York Times* about deep sleep secreting a chemical that's antagonistic to fibromyalgia (a muscular inflammation whose cause is not well understood) may be onto something important. When I took Halcion, another sleeping pill, my aches would increase, and next morning I would have the feeling somebody was causing them, and I would beome angry and keep thinking, "Who's doing this to me?"

I had never been inside the relatively new Radiation Oncology Center of the King City Medical Center. It had been "out there," a mysterious and somewhat frightening place for "unfortunate" people, a place I occasionally passed in my goings to and from the hospital or to one or more of the doctors practicing in its vicinity. Now *I* was one of the "unfortunates," about to become intimately acquainted with it. And its nurses and technicians and, above all, one of its radiation oncologists were to become intimately acquainted with *me*. It was a humbling role change, which I was by no means sure I would handle well. Yet I had a strong sense it was important to handle it well, that handling it well was an essential part of my healing process; that, indeed, I was a partner with the medical people in the success or failure of my therapy.

MARCH 11, 1993. When I had lunch today with a dermatologist friend, I told him about my Cibachrome printing interest and my prostate cancer experience. Like my friend John Lowrance, he said he was surprised I wasn't depressed, adding that I was in an excellent mood, and was "bringing intellect to bear" on my cancer situation. Although I was pleased to hear his comments,

I was afraid they were exaggerated, so I took them with the proverbial grain of salt. But he may have been right, for I was high at lunch, and afterwards I was eager to meet my radiation oncologist, Dr. Edward North, to discover the world of X-ray therapy and what was in store for me.

I had my first meeting, an orientation conference, with Dr. North this afternoon. It occurred in a small exam room of the solidly built, pleasant surroundings of the Oncology Center. He was in his mid-thirties, tall, intelligent, articulate, with an outgoing smile, a strong voice, and a short dark beard that contrasted with his white coat. A Phi Beta Kappa at Johns Hopkins, he had been a resident at a prominent medical school, where he had taught. He had published papers on prostate cancer, some recently.

"I'm a writer, and am interested in any information you can give me," I said.

"I'll give you more than you can probably handle," he responded with a smile, eyes bright with energy and goodwill.

"What would happen if I ignored my cancer?" I asked.

"You'd develop major problems—at first locally, then over wider areas. You wouldn't achieve your actuarial lifespan, which for somebody of your age is about eight to ten years. Very recent studies show that radiation therapy and surgery may be equal modalities for a fifteen-year survival rate."

I learned I'll have three planning sessions and thirty-eight X-ray treatments. The latter will occur Monday through Friday and will last seven and a half weeks. I was relieved to learn I'll be able to housesit for the Kenezes in California in July. I'll be finished with radiation therapy by then.

"The planning sessions are important. They'll customize your X-ray therapy," he said. "Four lead blocks the shape of your radiation fields will be made, and will be attached to the X-ray machine at the appropriate times. The first planning session will be a simulation one, during which a catheter will be inserted into your bladder and a tube into your rectum. You'll have another

CAT scan then. And a number of dots will be permanently tatooed on your hips and abdomen. Our goal is to have pictures showing the exact location of your prostate. Once the planning sessions are over, radiation technicians will administer the X rays. All the salient data (X-ray strength, time of exposure, location of the gland, and so on) will be digitized and fed into a computer, which will control much of the mechanics of therapy. If a technician should make a mistake, the computer will refuse to proceed. The X rays will be aimed at you from four directions: front, back and sides."

I'll be treated with X rays whose energy is 15 MV (15 million electron volt photons). The energy and wavelength of such X rays are similar to those of gamma rays. The difference is in the source. The X rays stem from a beam of electrons, produced by a linear accelerator (also called a linac), that strikes a tungsten target. (The linear accelerator is mounted in a gantry. The gantry rotates on a stand containing electronic and other systems.) Gamma rays, originating in atomic nuclei, are the product of radioactivity.

(Two or three weeks later I learned that before the introduction of megavoltage radiation [energies above 400,000 electron volts], skin damage often occurred, particularly in sensitive areas like the breasts. Also, bone absorbed radiation some three times more effectively than soft tissue, and as a consequence there was sometimes spontaneous fracture of bone.)

"How can the X rays differentiate between benign cells and cancer cells?" I asked.

"Good question. The DNA of the benign cells knows how to tell the cells to recover each day from the 'shove' of the X rays. For reasons not known, the DNA of the cancer cells doesn't know how to tell the cancer cells to do the same. So the benign cells recover, but the cancer cells don't."

"What about the possibility of incontinence as a result of radiation therapy?"

"Incontinence isn't normally one of the side effects of radiation. However, ulceration of the tip of the bladder and of the rectum *is* a possibility. If ulceration occurs, the tissues usually recover in several weeks. If they don't, surgery may be necessary. The first couple of weeks, you probably won't have any side effects. Later you may feel tired and have some diarrhea. Do you still achieve an erection?"

"Yes."

"Good. The chances of your losing that ability because of radiation are small. If you lose it, it will probably be through other causes. . . . Nature."

"There are plenty of other things I'm interested in."

He studied me across the great age gulf between us. "If you're not afraid of death, you're not afraid of impotence," he said.

I liked him very much, and felt I was in good hands. I had a hunch we were going to hit it off, and that I was taking an important step in my healing process.

"What are Gleason numbers?" I asked.

"Donald Gleason was a pathologist who worked at VA hospitals. Studying a large number of prostate biopsies available to him, he described major and minor patterns of cancer cells and assigned each a number from 1 to 5. The two patterns represent the degree of cancer cell aggressiveness. A patient's total number is the sum of the two patterns, the lowest being 2 and the highest 10. Gleason was able to predict the likely outcome of prostate cancers. If your Gleason score is 2 or 3 and you're along in years, you may have the option of safely ignoring the cancer, because you'll probably die of something else before the cancer gets you. If you have a 10, your chances of a cure are marginal, because this cell is very aggressive and may already have left the gland by the time you have your first biopsy. Yours is 6, in the middle. There's good reason to believe you'll be cured, and have the normal actuarial lifespan for a person your age."

After our talk, Dr. North examined my eyes and mouth; palpated the glands under my armpits; thumped parts of my back; listened to my chest with a stethoscope while ordering me to breathe in, breathe out; and palpated my abdomen and groin. Then he gave me a digital exam while I rested my elbows on the end of a gurney. I had had many digitals over the years, and they didn't bother me much any more. But the present one, the first after the biopsy (the tissues through which the needle had lunged were still supersensitive) was very unpleasant.

While doing it he remarked, "Ah. . . . I feel what Dr. Gilroy felt. The left lobe bulges toward the left. . . . Maybe 2 centimeters. The right lobe feels almost small."

I had felt robbed because my tumor or tumors lacked discrete form. I had wanted them to be like everybody else's (everybody being my cousins Erik and Murray). So now I was glad to imagine the left lobe bulging; to believe my cancer had some form, wasn't entirely amorphous. As I pulled up my trousers, I sensed a dripping from the end of my penis.

"What's wrong with the cancer cell's DNA?" I wondered as I drove homeward. "Why is it stupid? Is it so used to devastating the benign cells that it has become careless, hubristic? Has it forgotten that if you're going to wage war you'd better be prepared for a counterattack? Why has it overlooked the possibility of the benign cells having some friends out there? Maybe these geniuses of replication, these prostate cancer cells, are so busy replicating they haven't energy and concentration left over for defending themselves against radiation from what might feel to them is coming from outer space. You keep knocking a prostate cancer cell until its head falls off. I wonder if that delights the nearby benign cells, though they may be sick from their own knocks on the head."

HIV (human immunodeficiency virus) is much more clever than the prostate cancer cell. Knock HIV on the head with a drug and it promptly mutates. HIV doesn't bother to localize its activities, it's like a melanoma (an often deadly form of skin cancer) on the loose. But then HIV is a retrovirus, a form of life, or something between life and nonlife, whereas the prostate cancer cell is probably due to an error in the genetic command structure.

By the time I reached home, nerves were jangling throughout my body as a result of the digital.

"How did it go?" asked Joan.

"I lucked out!" I replied enthusiastically, despite the pain. "I have a great young oncologist!" And I described Dr. North.

"That's wonderful!" she cried. "You look tired. Get off your feet. Rest in the lounger."

I followed her advice. The jangling stopped only after she went out into the night and fetched a delicious Chinese dinner and a bottle of my favorite vodka. Tired, I turned in at 9:15. While undressing, I discovered some blood on my undershorts.

Next day, my friend Peter Kenez, gifted with irony, including self-irony, called from Aptos, California, in response to my letter informing him of my prostate cancer, and asked for details. I offered some. "Well, yesterday afternoon my oncologist gave me a digital exam," I added. "Coming after a biopsy, it wasn't pleasant. If anybody tells you it's nothing, don't believe it."

"Oy! Oy!" he responded in an agonized tone. "And now my sad story. Dorothy is dying." I knew Dorothy Dalby, his mother-in-law.

"From what?"

"She's in her mid-eighties, and she says she doesn't want to live any more."

"Is she sick?"

"Congestive heart failure. Life has become difficult. She has decided to die by not eating or drinking. Penny says no Jew would do that, it's a Gentile way to go. [Peter, a professor of Soviet History at the University of California at Santa Cruz, had been born Jewish in Hungary. Penny, his wife, a family therapist, had been born Gentile in the United States. I should perhaps note that I too was born Jewish and married a Gentile. And that I'm an Honorary Fellow of Peter's college, Adlai Stevenson.] So it's hard on us. We visit Dorothy, we chat, and she asks questions as if nothing unusual is going on. What's happening in Russia? Will Boris Yeltsin survive? How's the dog? How's my class? She'll die dreadfully, in great pain."

"I doubt it. She'll probably die of dehydration. Major organs will collapse."

"It will take her a month to die."

"That long?"

"It's so sad, but what can we do? Her daughter is coming from Australia. Grandchildren are arriving. And she's absolutely calm. No fear of death whatsoever. She's just tired of living."

"Why should she go on living if she's not enjoying it?"

"Probably her mind will go as she continues to starve. There will be dreadful scenes."

"My guess is that her mind will hold up well. And that there won't be dreadful scenes. She'll die suddenly."

"Well, what can one do? She's a real Gentile. No whining."

"Don't underestimate the Jews. They're not whiners either."

"Oy oy! You'll hear such whining when my time comes."

"I don't believe it, Peter. Peter, I miss you very much."

"I miss you too. We're getting older, Charles. It's important to hold on to friends."

My good mood was continuing. I was looking forward to my Cibachrome class tomorrow morning, and was worried because of news that a big snowstorm was coming, which might mean the class would be canceled. Printing in Cibachrome (full, rich color touted as being fade-resistant) had for me some of the adventure of fishing in a fast-flowing mountain stream or lake. Working in total darkness, carrying the wet unseen print from darkness into what felt at times like total light, I often wondered in suspense what I had caught. Caught, that is, in terms of a print. I wasn't in doubt about the quality of the original Antarctic image captured with a Leica on the Kodachrome slide. Would it be exciting, a keeper? Or disheartening, another failure, stealing the wind out of my sails?

The storm came, in the form of a huge snow blizzard, with high winds, and all classes were canceled at Mercer County Community College. Joan and I were snowed in. But I was glad, in a way, to stay home and work at writing. Meanwhile I was receiving calls from friends and relatives who wanted to know how I was doing and who, worried, wanted to buck me up. I was glad to be able to say, "No sweat. So far, so good. I brood occasionally, but that's natural, given my situation. On the whole, I'm doing well." I had no inkling of what was to come when I hit the hard times of radiation treatment.

MARCH 18, 1993. It was 12 degrees this morning. Joan couldn't get her car door open, so I went out and pried it loose. The door frame had frozen to the body. Dr. North said he'll numb the catheterization today, when he'll do a simulation (sim) session with me, but I'm apprehensive, probably because the only time I had a catheterization it was very unpleasant. This was at Dr. Gilroy's office a couple of years ago. I hadn't been told it was going to happen, and there was bleeding in my urine afterwards, followed by a combination of cystitis and prostatitis. (In a catheterization, a tube is inserted into the penis and the urethra and into the bladder.) I understand that not everyone has a strong reaction to a catheterization. Maybe the opening of my penis and of my urethra is not as large as other people's.

I entered the Radiation Oncology Center and then the men's dressing room, which contained small stalls with curtains, lockers with keys, and a toilet. A tall, stout, gray-haired, light-brown man was about to enter the latter.

41

"How are you?" he asked me.

"Fine!"

"*You're* cheerful. That's the main thing," he said as he disappeared behind the toilet door.

I undressed from the waist down, put on a hospital gown, and went to the waiting room. A woman in her thirties, with long blonde hair, came in, sat down, and asked me, "What kind of morning did you have?"

"Good!"

"Mine was terrible, terrible!" she said passionately.

Gluing her eyes to mine, she related her story. It was a forty-five-minute drive from her home to here. Instead of having her babysitter come today, she decided to leave her two kids, three and five, with a friend some miles away. Her car doors were frozen this morning. While she struggled to open the driver's door, her son, three, cried, tugging at her. Her hands were freezing. She was becoming desperate. She was going to be late for her therapy. She screamed at him, got the door open by pouring hot water over it, delivered her kids, and started for the hospital. Her rear car doors popped open. Parking her car on a shoulder, she tried to close them. They balked. Nobody stopped to help her, so she drove to a Texaco station, where a man fixed them with a hair dryer and squirts of silicon lubricant. He charged her $10.

"Ten dollars!" she cried. "Can you believe it? It took him ten minutes! What could I do? I paid!"

She was called away now. A nurse, saying "Drink this," handed me a medium-size styrofoam cup brimming with a very thick milk-white liquid. "Barium?" I asked. She left without answering.

Dr. North, smiling, appeared in the doorway. "I'm ready for you. Come with me," he said. I followed him into the small exam room in which we had conferred a week ago.

"I'll insert a catheter into your bladder today. And a tube into your rectum. And you'll be tattooed," he explained.

"Was that barium I drank?"

"Yes. It'll light up your intestines so I can block them from the treatment beam."

Red laser beams, part of today's procedure (they'll be used to pinpoint my therapy X rays), crisscross the simulation room. He holds up a piece of cardboard to show me two beams intersecting. They're beautiful; so pure a red; they make the imminent procedure less threatening. Their effect on me is therapeutic, maybe because, years ago, I imagined just such beams in self-hypnosis sessions that removed an unsightly growth from my left eye's lower lid.

"What did they do before lasers?" I ask.

"Guessed," he replies drily.

He instructs me to lie on a table.

"This is Joyce," he says.

"I can't see her from here."

"She's twenty months pregnant."

"We've met," says Joyce.

"I don't think so," I say.

"We have," Joyce insists.

"Where?"

Silence.

"Where?" asks Dr. North.

"I gave him the barium drink."

"This is Christina," says Dr. North.

"Hi, Christina," I say.

"Mr. Neider is a writer," says Dr. North. "He's very interested in our work." A silence. "I put a medication on the catheter. It will numb your penis. But at first it will burn a little."

As he begins inserting the instrument, the tip of my penis burns as if with an acid. The farther the catheter goes in, the deeper I feel the burning. I feel I'm being tortured. I hold my breath as my body wants to writhe. One of the nurses is holding my feet down.

43

In all the pain of it (for me) he asks, "How're you doing compared to being stranded in Antarctica?"

I had briefly told him, during our previous meeting, about my experience on Mount Erebus. I crack up with laughter.

"There's some blood," he says. I imagine it, and I imagine the catheter sliding into my bladder. The burning slowly subsides.

"Lift your knees," he instructs.

Joyce places a pillow under them. He thrusts a tube into my rectum.

"Clasp your hands on your chest," says Christina. "Breathe normally. But lie very still."

My feet are banded together. My hands are clasped on my chest. Unlike the time when, half-asleep, I was on the table for the bone scan, I'm hard awake, at times angry. I want the procedure to stop. The pain in my penis lessens, but I'm still aware of it, and I vividly remember the sensations of the catheter entering me. I feel wounded, vulnerable, needy. I stiffen at the thought of the pain that's coming when the catheter is removed. At the same time I admire a pattern of extremely small ruby dots made by a laser beam on the machine above me, and I notice with pleasure a rectangular hole in the ceiling's soundproofing, through which a ruby laser is shining.

"Are there four lasers in the room?" I ask.

"One, two . . . yes, four," says Christina, who I sense is young, with short hair, but whom I can't really make out from my elevated table in the room's dimness.

Why is the procedure taking so long? What are Christina and Joyce doing? Where's Dr. North? Can't they speed things up? Do they understand how uncomfortable it is to lie so still for so long with gadgets up your penis and rectum? My legs are trembling. Will relaxing them cause my body to move, spoiling the simulation? Letting the right one go just a bit, I'm surprised by how little it moves. The band around my feet is doing a good job. There's a windowed room on my left. I see a female figure moving around there. Occasionally a woman comes into the simulation room to make adjustments and to insert and remove photographic film plates. Twice Christina comes in to mark my hips. How long can I keep my hands clasped?

"These wash off," she says. "But the tattoos are permanent."

Dr. North, on my left, comes to say, "The four plates are excellent!"

I'm glad to see him. Though tall, he now looks amusingly short. I hadn't realized my table was so elevated.

At last the procedure seems over. There's only the tattooing left.

"How long did it take?" I ask Joyce, who's somewhere on my right.

"About an hour."

"Do you think the discomfort of a catheter is as hard for females as for males?"

"I think *so*."

Finally free to unclasp my hands, I have trouble moving my fingers. Joyce tattoos me. I expected only two or three tattoo dots. I get nine. She stabs, then wipes blood away.

"Joyce, how about tattooing a little heart on my hip?"

"That costs a lot extra."

The worst of the three planning sessions is over. Next Tuesday I'll have a CAT scan, but without drinking lots of liquid, and without an IV. This will be followed by an interval of two weeks during which my customized equipment will be made. Finally, I'll be filmed to check that my blocks were made exactly as specified, and that I'll receive the correct radiation doses. Meanwhile I'll rest and heal, as I did after the biopsy. Side effects will come only after the radiation. However, such reassuring thoughts fail to diminish my present discomfort and fatigue. I want to go home and close my eyes.

Instead, I go to the toilet to urinate. Blood. Pain. I wipe my behind to remove the lubrication used in inserting the rectal tube. A feeling of great messiness.

Glancing at the spotless mirror, I'm startled. My lips are fiercely white, like those of a mime or clown. Result of the barium drink. The white is recalcitrant; only hard work with water and a paper towel removes it. I slowly get dressed, feeling as if somebody hit me in the balls with a baseball bat.

"What twists and turns we mortals endure. But what high technology some of us lucky ones have available!" I tell myself, and think of the millions of people in our country without health insurance, and of the many in other nations who have nothing.

Reporting to Dr. North's office, I tell him I was catheterized only once before, and that I got both cystitis and prostatitis out of it and needed to take antibiotics. His dark eyebrows go up in surprise.

"Would it be useful for me to take antibiotics as a precautionary measure?" I ask.

"I'm glad you told me. I'll give you four Cipros. Take them twice daily."

"When will I begin X-ray therapy?"

"Early April."

"Why do you suppose my cousin Murray had thirty or thirty-two treatments, whereas I'll have thirty-eight?"

"Doctors don't get sued if there's no cure. They get sued for side effects. The more rads [radiation absorbed dosage] you give, the greater the chance of a cure; also, a higher percentage of side effects. So doctors tend to be very conservative. I'm still innocent, I still go by the literature. I try hard for a cure. It's a combination of philosophy and biology."

As I left the Oncology Center, my penis, urethra, bladder, and rectum insistently told me they hated gravity. At home I sat in a lounger and tried to keep my mind off my body. Hours after the catheterization there was still a terrible burning in the opening of my penis during urination, and it was very painful to start and stop. In addition, my rectum and anus were sore. My whole groin felt very sensitive, and heavier than usual.

"Have you looked at your tattoos?" Joan asked me about an hour later.

"I have such a pot that I can't see beyond it."

"No, you don't!" she said, laughing.

The tattoo marks were more numerous than I had expected. I had eleven, not nine: three on my left hip, four on my right, four on my abdomen.

Four

March 23 to April 10, 1993

MARCH 23, 1993. Cousin Erik called today, and we got to talking about Dr. Fledermaus, his urologist. "I'm angry about him," I said. "He talked you into a radical prostatectomy. And rushed you into it. He's a shvitzer. [Literally, someone who sweats; who's on the run.] And a money-grabber. If it turns out your Gleason number was very low, you ought to sue him for malpractice."

A low Gleason score, particularly at Erik's age (seventy-one) when his prostate cancer was diagnosed, would have suggested the advisability of watchful waiting; or, at any rate, of conservative radiation therapy. I had no hesitation in speaking boldly to him. He was my relative. Also, I loved him—he was intelligent, cultured, sensitive, charming, physically strong, and had a wild sense of humor that had given me many a belly laugh, so much so that it had often reduced me to tears. It was a sense of humor that was conspicuously and painfully lacking during his long recovery from the prostatectomy, when, despite warm support from family and friends, he was often depressed.

And—and this was important, as I was beginning to understand—we were both members of the same club, a cancer club; in particular, the prostate cancer club; and as club members we had the right, even the duty, to speak to the point. Still, this wasn't entirely true, for in certain instances being club members didn't necessarily encourage (or permit) frank discussion of a potentially painful subject. For example, with Cousin Murray I had to be more or less closemouthed. I had to walk on eggshells, because he didn't care to talk about his prostate cancer, or about any topic closely associated with it. Or maybe he didn't want to talk about them with *me*.

"Fledermaus has two young kids," said Erik defensively. "I wouldn't want to risk ruining his career. But I'll definitely ask him for my Gleason number when I see him on June 10."

"June 10 is a long way off," I said. Erik let this remark go by him. "Remember," I said, "he didn't warn you that removal of your lymph nodes might lead to enormously swollen testicles. [We'll hear more about this later.] And he failed to advise you to wear a suspensory to protect your scrotum. Remember how horrified you were, and how much suffering you had to endure. Fledermaus's two young kids have nothing to do with it. He probably harmed you, and may be harming other people, and should be prevented from doing it."

Erik groaned, but said nothing more on the subject. I had the feeling I had overstated my case and was being harsh on the subject of Dr. Fledermaus, and possibly cruel. But it was too hard to resist saying what I had said to Erik, whose suffering, as a consequence of the radical prostatectomy, I had witnessed at first hand and at length, both in the hospital and in his home. I think, having selected radiation, I was high on it, as if I had escaped a prostatectomy; and this high was buttressd by my high on Dr. Edward North, whom I greatly admired and who believed in the virtues and rewards of radiation. Also, I was high on the Radiation Oncology Center (the physical plant) and on the employees with whom I had come in contact there.

And yet, despite my high, there was always the basic question, beating like an ominous drum: Would the radiation work—for *me*? What if the answer was No!? It was suspense I would have to live with for some time. My PSA three or four months after the completion of radiation would be the first significant clue.

My mind was full of ferment. Joan laughed when I said there were currently four exhibitions at the Metropolitan Museum of Art I wanted to see: a Greek one ("The Greek Miracle," in the Lehman wing); a Daumier one, which had received wonderful reviews; a history of photography (the first century); and a Havemeyer exhibition ("Splendid Legacy"). At the same time, I seemed to be more worried about my Cibachrome prints, about which I lay awake occasionally, thinking about filtration, exposure, and chemistry, than about my cancer. Was this a displacement?

This week I read the government publication *Radiation Therapy and You: A Guide to Self-Help During Treatment* (NIH Publication No. 91-2227, revised October 1990), given to me by the Radiation Oncology Center. It listed many possible side effects. Some might occur regardless of what part of the body was irradiated: emotional changes due to fatigue and to effects on hormones; lowered blood counts; lowered immune system; changes in skin sensitivity; loss of appetite. Others were related to the part of the body being treated. With treatment of the abdominal and pelvic regions the following were possible: nausea, diarrhea, frequent and uncomfortable urination. (There were other possible side effects for women, such as vaginal dryness, with consequent painful intercourse.) I wondered if I would have any or many of the side effects mentioned in the book, and why Cousin Murray had had none.

I had a CAT scan today to determine exactly where my prostate is located. The purpose: precise aiming of X rays. When I arrived at the Oncology Center, Cybill, a brunette radiation technology therapist, told me to get undressed and handed me a cotton hospital robe to wear over my hospital gown. After changing I went to the oncology waiting room, where I saw a posted notice: Prostate Cancer Support Group, for men with or recovering from prostate cancer. Next meeting: March 31 at the Franklin House in King City.

Wanting to know as much as possible about prostate cancer, and thinking I could do worse than learn about it from men who had it, I resolved to join the group. A group of men wishing to support each other. But whom could I, a tenderfoot, support? Men who had walked down the dark road. Maybe some who were still walking down it. Would they all be graybeards? And would I be the oldest?

Soon afterwards Cybill led me to the nuclear medicine part of the hospital, where I read a magazine while she changed the sheets on the CAT scan table.

A man in his fifties, with blond hair and wearing a hospital gown, was being wheeled past me. "Good luck!" he said heartily, raising his right thumb.

Smiling, I raised mine silently. He laughed. I wondered if he was laughing at our common fate.

Cybill took me to the table, arranged me on it, and attached three fine, blue-white catheter tubes, each about an inch long, to my skin with tape, then left the room to make the exposures. I waited while she developed and examined the films.

Returning, she said, "You'll get your third planning session in about two and a half weeks."

"I'm making progress!" I thought, impatient to begin radiation and come to grips with my cancer. In particular, I wanted to know where I'd stand by May 7, when I was scheduled to attend an Antarctic workshop, sponsored by the National Science Foundation, in Boulder, Colorado.

MARCH 27. I've been feeling "down" the past three or four days—tired and distracted. Why? Is this related to my having cancer? Yesterday was almost a spring day. I should have walked, but didn't. But today I did—the first full walk in two weeks.

Questions, questions. When will my therapy start? At what time of day will it be given? If I had a full-time job would my treatments be scheduled accordingly? Will I have minor side effects? Major? Appetite trouble? Diarrhea? Will I be able to continue my power walks, or will I be obliged to change to slower, shorter ones? Will the radiation affect my behavior during the coming trip to Boulder? What will my PSA be after radiation therapy? Will it return to what it was before it rose to 14.4 and then to 16.4? Will it again be high, reflecting a benign enlargement of the gland, or will it drop into the normal range, 1 to 4?

I'm impressed by the behavior of all the women I've encountered at the hospital. They're wonderful: bright, eager to help, articulate, knowledgeable, almost affectionate. The only man I've dealt with so far is Dr. North, and he's wonderful too. It must sound ridiculous to an outsider (a healthy person, one not in need of hospitals and frequent visits to doctors), but so far it's almost a pleasure for me to go to the Medical Center.

I called the number listed for the support group and spoke with Harry Stengel, the leader, who welcomed me into the group, which meets once a month.

"Has your cancer metastasized?" he asked.

I had a twinge of guilt before replying, "No."

Was I going to be feeling guilty in the group because I was a newcomer to cancer? Probably. But being a newcomer wasn't my fault, any more than my cancer was my fault. But if my cancer wasn't *my* fault, whose fault was it? God's? Society's? My diet? My age? My gender? My testosterone? Braking this stream of thought, I was surprised to find myself involved in such idiotic questions, questions that from time to time seemed naturally to accompany my new companion: my cancer.

MARCH 31, 1993. Rain, rain, dreary rain the past couple of days. I joined the King City prostate cancer support group today. Cousin Murray's wife, Jan, on hearing I planned to join the group, had remarked to Murray, "What does he want to join a support group for? It'll only depress him." Which

Murray had repeated to Erik, and Erik had repeated to me. Erik said Jan and Murray believe in knowing as little as possible about Murray's cancer and the treatment for it, because that's what they're comfortable with; and they dislike discussing cancer in general, as well as his in particular. It should be remembered that Murray, according to his and Jan's account, had no side effects in his radiation therapy; that is, if one omits his probable impotence.

There are currently twenty-two members in the King City support group. Present today, in addition to myself, were four men and a woman. The woman was the spouse of one of the men. Yes, I was easily the oldest person present at this meeting, and perhaps the most fit, physically. The setting was formal, a beautiful, large room in a stone house, but we were tieless, and we addressed each other by our first names. Harry Stengel, a genial, soft-spoken, white-haired man with a pleasant smile, began the session by announcing that one member was in the hospital, a second was attending a funeral, and a third was very sick. What a beginning for a newcomer, I thought. It was almost enough to frighten him away.

Stengel mentioned a member, with recurrence of bleeding from his penis, who had had a PSA of 5000, but whose PSA had dropped to 80 or 90 after some treatment. (Stengel didn't say which kind.) He said the member swears by shark cartilage though it's very expensive, because sharks don't have cancer (so the member believes).

"I've heard there's no limit to how high a PSA can go," said Pete Wayne casually, sitting on my left.

I was stunned by the figure of 5000 for a PSA, I who had been shocked by my 16.4. I hadn't imagined a PSA could go that high. It was like reading in the *New York Times* about the discovery of a black hole (in a neighboring galaxy) with a mass of 3 billion suns. Or could the 5000 have been an error of reporting? And the image of blood issuing from the absent member's penis pained me. I was indeed a tenderfoot in these matters. But this was all the more reason for becoming an integral part of the group. After all, I had told myself I wanted to learn a great deal about prostate cancer. So now I was learning about it.

When Harry Stengel asked me to introduce myself, I did so only in terms of my cancer, saying it was Stage B1, localized in one lobe, with a PSA of 16.4, a Gleason score of 6, and that I was waiting to begin a course of radiation therapy at the Radiation Oncology Center. No point, I thought, in boring strangers with anything more personal than that. I seemed to be right; I wasn't asked about anything more personal.

At Stengel's suggestion, a man named Davy Florence, saying he wouldn't be with us much longer because he was retiring to Florida, reported on his prostate cancer history. With a PSA of 55, he had had three separate biopsies, all negative. His internist, concerned about Florence's PSA, had urged him to have some tests, so Florence had had an MRI (magnetic resonance imaging), a bone scan and a CAT scan. They had revealed bone lesions, meaning the cancer had traveled to his bones. He had had an orchiectomy (surgical castration) to stop the formation of testosterone, a male hormone, in his testicles. Testosterone aids the cancer cells to replicate and spread. And he was taking flutamide (brand name Eulexin) to suppress the male hormone produced in his adrenals.

Again I was shocked, this time by the fact that Florence had had three biopsies, and that all had been negative, despite a PSA of 55. How could such a thing happen? Where had the cancer cells been hiding? And my *one* biopsy had been unpleasant enough. The thought of three. . . . I imagined Florence's mood swings . . . from anxiety to elation . . . to anxiety. . . . Though I wanted to know more about his experience with his cancer, I was too shy, as a newcomer, to ask him. What did his tale imply? Why hadn't his urologist urged him to get an MRI, a CAT scan, and a bone scan inasmuch as he had so high a PSA? Why was it left for his internist to make the suggestion? How long could his cancer be kept at bay?

We spoke about biopsies, and somebody asked if anyone had experienced bleeding from the penis afterwards. All but Harry Stengel said they had.

I said, "I asked my urologist, Dr. Lewis Gilroy, if such bleeding, if it comes from the prostate, can spread cancer cells beyond the gland. He said he seriously doubts it."

"It's very reassuring to hear you say that," said Davy Florence, looking gratefully at me. "It's something I've been thinking about. These meetings *are* very useful. I've learned some important things."

I wondered why he hadn't asked his urologist the same question.

"Get used to it all being relative," I told myself. "His cancer has spread to his bones. And he has lost his testicles. Yet he's reassured that the bleeding from his penis hasn't spread the cancer to tissues beyond the gland."

I told myself I had a lot to learn from this group; and that much of the learning would be painful; that I had to get used to it, but without hardening myself; and that I was—so far (knock on wood!)—remarkably lucky by comparison. Also, that I should accept my guilt feelings as normal; and that, down the road, I might encounter hard times that might make *this* time seem a blessedly innocent one.

A beeper in Harry Stengel's pocket went off. He pulled out an ivory-looking little case, turned the sound off, and downed a pill with the help of water in a small plastic bottle he carried with him. A little later a similar device beeped in Davy Florence's pocket, and Florence swallowed a pill dry.

"It's for my hot flashes," said Florence.

"At these meetings there's a good deal of beeping going on," whispered Pete Wayne to me with a distant, ironic smile.

"Hot flashes?" I asked Florence.

"It's because of my orchiectomy," he explained in a mild tone. He was a mild-mannered man, and the only one at the meeting who wore a full suit. I wondered if he was a retired academic. "It's because I have no testicles. I'm going through male menopause. I take a special pill twice daily for the hot flashes. And I avoid milk. I have the sensation I'm getting cold before the flash comes on. I try to ignore it. The flash lasts about two minutes. Sometimes I break out into a heavy sweat."

"I too am in male menopause," said Harry Stengel. "I'm on Lupron [leuprolide]. Hormone therapy. It's medical castration."

"Are you on anything else?" I asked.

"Just flutamide. I have bone lesions. Hormone therapy isn't a cure. It's suppressive therapy," said Stengel with a wry smile, glancing around the room.

"How do you take the Lupron?" I asked.

"By injection. Once a month. It's expensive. But I'm covered by insurance."

Then a man named John Darrough, who spoke in a high voice and with a slightly foreign-sounding accent, and who became increasingly excited as he spoke, eyes flashing and shoulders growing tense, told about the death of his younger brother about a year ago. And how the brother had had a radical prostatectomy in his early fifties that had left him impotent. And how, some ten years later, the brother had remarked to John Darrough, "I didn't realize until recently that the prostate operation did that to me!"

"And he was single!" said John Darrough hotly, almost shouting. "The operation changed his life!"

I thought, "Why didn't his brother ask his urologist or some other doctor what had caused his impotence? Was he timid? Embarrassed? But this was his life, the only one that had been allotted to him!"

But I said nothing, having decided that this was my listening day, mainly.

"A friend of mine hates all urologists," said Harry Stengel with a smile.

The woman, John Darrough's wife, said nothing during the meeting, but her gaze was keen, and I gathered she was absorbing everything. I liked her, and I liked John Darrough, and I liked Harry Stengel, with his very gentle manner. Later in this narrative there will be an interview with Stengel, and one with the Darroughs.

APRIL 2, 1993. To make sure I had gotten it right, that Davy Florence hadn't meant three specimens instead of three biopsies, I called him this morning and checked it out with him.

"I had three separate and negative biopsies," he said. "The biopsies were done by two urologists. My original urologist was away at one point. About a year intervened between biopsies. Cancer was never detected in my prostate."

"That's extraordinary! What happened to it?"

"I don't know. Your guess is as good as mine."

"Did any of your doctors speculate about it?"

"Not to my knowledge."

"Did you ask?"

"No. I guess it seemed beside the point. I had cancer, and that was *it*."

"But how could the two urologists *and* the pathologists have failed to find the original cancer, the cancer in the site of origin?"

"You can fool *me*. The answer probably is that they still don't have a good handle on prostate cancer. The orchiectomy [by the way, this word and *orchid* stem from the Greek word for testicle] was a simple operation, done in a morning. The healing process took eight or nine days. I should have been put on flutamide some weeks prior to the operation, but for some reason wasn't. My internist recently told me my PSA is 'below measurable.'"

"How come the two urologists didn't urge you to have the bone and CAT scans?"

"I don't know. Other people have wondered about it."

"Who's your internist?"

"Daniel Redmont. He insisted I get the tests. I like him. I believe in him."

"I do too."

"He may have saved my life. The last time he did a digital on me he said, 'I can't believe how much this thing has shrunk.' I may have been living with this cancer for some time. I have a couple of hot spots in my bone. One is between my shoulder blades. I sometimes wonder if it came from playing football many years ago."

There was a long pause.

"I'd like my testicles back . . ." he said wistfully.

That really hit me in the gut. Poor guy, he had been through the mill. But at least he was still alive—and kicking. I wondered how well I would do in his shoes. Cancer relativity. I was happy my cancer hadn't left the gland. Harry Stengel was happy he hadn't lost his testicles. Davy Florence was happy his cancer hadn't spread beyond his bones. Other people were happy their cancer hadn't gone into their lungs or liver.

APRIL 6, 1993. A note from Peter Kenez today informed me that his mother-in-law, Dorothy Dalby, died very peacefully on March 26.

I have an appointment tomorrow for my third and final planning session. I've been told that if all goes well, I may begin my treatment then. I'm excited by the idea of starting, being able to look ahead and gauge how I'll be doing by May 7, when I'm to go to Boulder for the Antarctic conference. Susy, my daughter, said she'd like to go with me when I have my first treatment.

"It's important to have someone come with you, to hold your hand," she said.

"If you want to come, I won't say no," I said. "But if you think I'm anxious, I'm not. Actually, I'm eager to begin. Nothing invasive will occur. I won't feel anything. It'll take a while for side effects to show up, if they do."

"I agree it isn't necessary. But if you change your mind. . . ."

My friend John Lowrance thinks I should let her come with me, at least once.

"It would be good for your relationship," he said. "Don't be rational about it. It's not a rational matter."

"The reason I'm approaching this business with some equanimity is my age," I said. "I've used up most of my life. I have little to lose."

I think Susy offered to come with me because she knew Joan probably wouldn't, and that I certainly wouldn't expect Joan to. It wasn't that Joan wasn't empathetic toward me. It was simply that she and I were used to doing many things apart from each other.

I recall an incident that may throw some light on my relationship with Joan. It occurred in 1976 shortly before I left the States on my third Antarctic trip. I had noticed that people who knew I was heading for Antarctica (and there was some local publicity about it) behaved in a maternal manner toward me. Preferring not to have a Navy haircut in the Antarctic, I went to get a haircut from a young Sicilian barber I knew well in Princeton. I always got a simple scissors cut from him, not a razor one, which was more expensive and elaborate. Without offering an explanation, he proceeded to give me a fancy razor one, yet charged me for a scissors cut. I was touched.

While I was in the chair, he suddenly asked, "How can you sleep when you're in Antarctica?"

I was puzzled. I wondered if he was referring to being able to sleep while the sun never sets. "What do you mean?" I asked.

He explained, "When I sleep, I sleep just so, with my leg across my wife's leg. If I didn't do that, I wouldn't be able to sleep."

I laughed. "Well, I don't have that strong a sleep habit," I said. "If I did, I probably wouldn't be able to go to the Antarctic."

Jan, Cousin Murray's wife, had accompanied him when he had gone for his radiation treatments, and had driven him home. And Barbara Darrough, as I learned from Harry Stengel, always attended support group meeings with her husband. Probably Murray and John Darrough were comfortable with that. I, on the other hand, preferred to be alone. It would have felt strange, almost like a burden, to know that someone was waiting for me, someone who probably would distract me from what else was going on around me.

I took my usual vigorous walk this morning. What will happen to the walk as I proceed with therapy? Will its length and pace decrease? Will I be forced to stop walking altogether? Two booklets about cancer advise wearing loose clothes during treatment, primarily to spare irradiated skin. Too late to reduce my waist. Will my trousers be too tight? Do I dare to eat a peach?

I'm scheduled to do some Cibachrome printing with strangers in a smaller lab about a week from now. What if I have diarrhea? After how many treatments does it usually occur? How frequent and urgent would the movements be? It would be embarrassing to have to leave the lab's total darkness several times, disturbing my fellow printers. What would they think? What explanation could I give?

APRIL 7, 1993. When I arrived at the Oncology Center for a 5:00 o'clock appointment for my Planning Session 3 (a filming) today, the lobby was empty. This was my first visit to the Oncology Center after lobby hours. I went to the little waiting room. There was no one around. It felt eery to be alone in the place. Had I made a mistake? Or had there been a mixup in my appointment time?

Hearing some papers being shuffled in a small area behind a wall, I presented myself to a female radiation therapy technician, who told me to change in the dressing room. The dressing room was empty, the bathroom door was ajar. All the lockers had keys in them, meaning they were free. Removing my trousers and undershorts and donning a green hospital gown,

I returned to the radiation station, where I felt very vulnerable in my hospital gown, open at the back. Was that a draft I was feeling in my crotch?

"You'll start treatment on Monday," said the technician. "What time would you like to select? These are still available."

She showed me a list. It was an exciting moment for me, the end of much suspense.

"2:15," I replied.

I was greeted by two young women in white, both named Marie. They were radiation therapy technologists, also called technicians. They led me to the nearby treatment room, which felt similar to the simulation room. I lay down on the extremely narrow treatment table, also known as the treatment couch. One of the Maries placed a white pillowcase across my loins, reached under it and lifted my hospital gown almost to my nipples.

"No point in worrying about modesty," I thought. "They've seen it all. And in men a great deal younger than you. And with much bigger equipment. So lie quietly and accept. Resignation's the thing here. Relax. Enjoy."

The other Marie strapped my feet together. My hands were immobile on my chest. Yanking carefully on the sheet beneath me and cautioning me not to try to cooperate, the Maries arranged my body by millimeters. Then, using ruby-colored lasers and my tattoo marks, they lined up the large radiation machine, inserted a customized block into the machine, and left the room to avoid being exposed to X rays, leaving me alone with the potentially murderous, potentially life-saving equipment as it buzzed. I thought, "So this is how it will feel when I get the actual radiation."

I felt I had come a long way from the time when I was looking at Dr. Gilroy's light screen and wondering, in great suspense, like someone charged with a serious crime, what the verdict in my case would be: if my cancer had invaded important soft tissues and/or bones. Well, it hadn't; and here I was, in this very modern room, being treated as if I had been innocent all along.

I was being zapped by X rays, but not with the strength I would receive during radiation therapy. The function of this filming session was to make sure the rays were being aimed with great precision. Studying the ceiling, I focused on a small rectangle cut in the soundproofing tiles, an edge of which showed a thin beam of laser light composed of millions of tiny ruby beads that seemed to be trembling for some quantum-mechanical reason.

I was comforted by their beauty and by the knowledge they were an important part of my treatment. In the presence of caring young women operating a complex machine, I felt so secure that at one point I fell into a soothing sleep. I was awakened by sounds made by one of the Maries as she adjusted the equipment.

"May I feel a block's heft?" I asked her.

She handed me a block. It had been screwed to a heavy plexiglas board containing many holes. It was heavy, but not as heavy as lead. The device is slipped and locked into place on a shelf beneath the treatment head (the X-ray aperture).

The Maries took four large films, called plates, from my front, back and sides, using a different customized block for each view. Silence while the films were being developed automatically by a machine in another room. My therapy environment was becoming familiar to me: machine, lasers, table, strapped feet, the fact that part of my groin was exposed. After the last zap, and while the Maries were still out of the room, I reached down to check how much of me was exposed. My abdominal/pelvic area was naked down to the base of my penis.

When it was time for me to sit up, I discovered with surprise that it wasn't easy for me to do so. Because of the narrowness of the treatment table, there was little to press my palms against. And, let's face it, my abdominal muscles weren't what they had once been. "Take it easy, you're in your late seventies," I reminded myself, as if it was possible to forget this strange fact. Momentarily irritated by the architecture of hospital gowns, I left the table awkwardly, feeling I was exposing myself.

"Sorry," I said. "I don't mean to be flashing. I don't normally flash."

"It's nothing to be embarrassed about," said the Marie with the long golden hair, whom I was beginning to like because of her warm, friendly manner. The other Marie was nice too, but cooler both in complexion and in manner. I called them Marie, they called me Mr. Neider. I still didn't know their last names. I felt grateful to them for making me feel very comfortable.

As I left the treatment room, somebody in white handed me a booklet, *Radiation Therapy and You*, and some papers. The papers, a stapled form of five sheets titled *Radiation Therapy Nursing Assessment*, contained many questions for me to answer. There were also three other sheets with these respective titles: *Information for Patients Getting Radiation to the Pelvis and Bladder; Instructions for Your Blood Tests;* and *Preventive Skin Care Guidelines While Undergoing Your Radiation Treatment.*

The dressing room felt strangely empty, as if it was all pleasantly mine and had nothing to do with disease and pain. I was no longer merely a potential customer. I had been admitted to the club of those undergoing radiation therapy. I was eager to look at a calendar to view time's layout. I would have an unvarying routine now, at least in mid-week.

APRIL 10, 1993. I was greatly impressed today by my granddaughter Annie's computer ability. She's not quite four!

Two more days before being zapped, having the rays go deep inside me. My inner body will be bathed by an energetic light, and an inner radiance will ensue.

When I was handed the questionnaire and the set of papers at the conclusion of the filming session the other day, I noticed that nurse Debby Kuban had, in writing, suggested soap I should use during X-ray therapy: Dove, Caress or Tone. (Normal soaps are too harsh for irradiated skin.) I bought four bars of unscented Dove. Yesterday morning I opened one of them.

By evening I realized it was so scented I wouldn't be able to use it. Last night I sealed the bar in a sandwich bag so the odor wouldn't disturb me during the night. Also, this would give me time to consider what to do. By morning the odor had penetrated the plastic.

Joan agreed the bar was heavily scented. What did the manufacturer mean by *unscented*? This morning I went to the market and studied the soap section. I saw no Tone. But there were several kinds of Caress. I bought one labeled "Lightly scented" although I could easily smell its perfume through the package. "Maybe it will be less scented than the unscented Dove," I thought.

At home I handed Joan the Caress. She agreed it was scented.

"It's scented even through the package," I said. "I wonder if the Dove is scented like that."

I fetched a packaged bar of Dove. No odor. I opened the package. Still no odor. The scented bar had been mistakenly packaged! Eureka! I was saved! Meanwhile Joan, bending over, was laughing. I opened the two other packages of Dove. No scent! Hooray!

I took a bar of Dove to my bathroom, removed the Ivory bar from the shower's built-in soap dish and placed the Dove bar in the dish. Returning to Joan, I said I would use Dove for my entire body, because there was only one soap dish in my shower. And why did nurse Debby Kuban, without being explicit, imply I should use Dove or Caress or Tone in my groin area, probably also in my crotch? After all, I wasn't going to be X-rayed in my crotch, was I, God forbid?

Again Joan laughed wildly.

Five

April 12 to April 24, 1993

APRIL 12, 1993. Treatment 1 of 38. While shaving, I think of being zapped today, and imagine the rays zapping me, then think it's not a good idea to use the word *zap*, which suggests body damage. Better to think of kindly rays, otherwise who knows what psychosomatic evil may result?

Consider the alternatives, I tell myself: surgery or doing nothing. Surgery: the dangers of general anesthesia; a long recovery time; maybe permanent incontinence; probable impotence. Doing nothing: the disease's inexorable course?

After showering this morning I start applying Zeasorb, an absorbent powder, to my groin, then remember the injunction against talcum powder. Talc contains metal, which intensifies the X rays' burning effect. Women being irradiated for breast cancer are advised to stop using underarm deodorants because the latter contain aluminum. Because I'm uncertain how much talcum Zeasorb contains, I wash the area and apply cornstarch, which is acceptable. No point in starting radiation with a little act of rebellion.

It was a beautiful day, 55 degrees and sunny. I had my usual walk. During four hours this morning I made five Cibachrome prints, then hurried for my first radiation treatment. A teenage girl with dark, thick hair was alone in the Oncology Center waiting room when I entered it. She smiled briefly at me before returning to her magazine. "You're too young to be in this kind of trouble," I thought. I wanted to say something friendly but decided it was best not to. Sitting down opposite her, I realized this wouldn't do unless I was willing to risk exposing myself. The hospital gown, which when I was standing seemed long enough, had hiked up to just below my knees; and, under the gown, I was naked from the waist down, except for shoes and socks. I disliked the idea of having to press my legs together to be decent; my thigh muscles weren't used to doing it.

The chair on her left was unused. Would she think I was pressing my luck if I lessened the distance between us by using the chair? Telling myself I had more important things to worry about, I decided to occupy it, and stood up and reached for a magazine.

At this moment a very small older woman with thinning brown hair entered the room, took the vacant seat and conversed in a low tone in Spanish with the teenager. My relations with hospital gowns suffered a setback, for I had no choice but to sit with legs together like a skirted Catholic-school girl. The woman wore a hospital gown and tiny athletic shoes. She seemed to have turned in on herself; to have become wizened by pain and anxiety.

Nurse Debby Kuban came in and spoke with the teenager in English. The teenager interpreted for the woman. "It happened at 2 A.M. Not too watery," said the teenager, smiling. Did she think it necessary to smile because, being in a hospital, she needed to ward off the evil eye? Normally I would have thought this elderly woman and I had nothing in common. (What was elderly? I was probably older than she.) Now, it seemed, we might have a good deal. What kind of radiation was she getting? Abdominal-pelvic? Would I too soon have diarrhea? "I'll give you some medicine," said Debby Kuban reassuringly to the teenager.

In the treatment room I asked for more pillows as I lay down on the patient's table. "You can't have it. This is the pillow you used during the simulation," said Joy Engelson, a blonde technician. "The process mustn't be varied." I had a pain in my right shoulder blade but there was nothing I could do about it. "Relax your bottom," said Marie Izant as she readied me for the X-ray machine.

"Why is it important to have a full bladder when coming to therapy?" I asked Marie Izant.

"When the bladder is distended it tends to move out of the X-ray field and therefore avoids being injured by the rays. You don't have to be on the verge of wetting yourself. And if you have to go, *go*."

The ceiling lights were turned off while the machine was being adjusted and aimed. They were turned on while I lay—alone—in the room, waiting for the prolonged buzzing that would indicate the rays were coming at me. The bright lights were unpleasant, made me want to shut my eyes, but I kept them open for some reason. I stared at the huge machine's marblelike arch above me, which showed haphazard black scratches.

Come, kindly light, murder the disease trying to murder me.

The buzzing began. I felt myself drifting off. The three lady technicians, who had been attending the control console outside the radiation room, reentered the room.

"What are the black scratches?" I asked Joy Engelson.

"Oh, they're due to our laziness," she replied with a laugh. I didn't bother to ask what she meant. How wonderfully tolerant of my questions these ladies were, how almost eager to please.

"I'm a very old party," said Somerset Maugham in his old age. Was he older than I am now?

"Don't step down yet, you're still high up," warned Joy Engelson as my session ended. I hadn't realized I had ascended.

Immediately after the treatment, I met with nurse Debby Kuban in one of the two small exam rooms and learned that the metal used for the blocks is Cerrobend, a lead alloy. A styrofoam mold is made; the Cerrobend is poured into it; and the block is finished by an in-house craftsman. My daily rad (radiation absorbed dose, as the reader will recall) is 180.

"You'll probably be able to continue your walks, but maybe after a while you'll do your three miles more slowly," Debby Kuban said. "It's okay to have sexual relations. You may lose some desire. A number of patients have reported they didn't keep an erection long. Some people prefer to know minimally. Others ask questions, they want to understand. We think the people who ask questions help their therapy by knowing what's happening."

I received several calls in the evening, among them one from Cousin Erik and another from my daughter Susy. Susy asked how my first session had gone.

I said, "Smoothly. I'm fascinated by the process. And I enjoy the help of the very pleasant and efficient young female technicians."

"Did they take your left testicle?" asked Susy jokingly. My relations with her had always been informal; and we had, a couple of days earlier, spoken about testicular cancer.

We laughed.

APRIL 13. Treatment 2 of 38. Today I wore a blue cotton gown over my hospital gown, which made it unnecessary for me to reach behind myself to tie the hospital gown, a procedure that sometimes irritated me. Just before today's treatment I spoke with nurse Tanya O'Neill, who said she had met me during my CAT scan. She was sitting with Debby Kuban at the curved high desk across the corridor from the waiting room.

"You probably won't feel fatigue until late in your therapy," she said. "In a couple of weeks you may have some bladder and bowel irritation."

"How long does it take for water to reach the bladder?" I asked.

"About twenty minutes."

"I swallowed a large cup and a half just before leaving home." I omitted mentioning I had had a shot of vodka with the water.

"That's perfect," she said, referring to the timing.

The four treatment fields are front, back, right side, left side. I'm given the treatment in that order. The patient's table ascends. The ceiling lights are partly obscured by the machine above me. The ladies leave the room. I hear a buzzing that lasts ten or twelve seconds. The ladies enter. The machine swivels to beneath me, exposing my eyes to the bright, circular ceiling lights. The first block is replaced by the second. The ladies leave the room. And so on. Almost before I know it, I'm finished. The ladies come in, my table slides away from the machine, descends, and I'm allowed to sit up and step down.

I've read that some patients are frightened by the machine; or rather the machinery. It *is* overpowering-looking. It's truly massive. And it makes loud noises: grunts, groans, and occasionally something that might, to a highly strung person, suggest a shriek. You can't help but wonder, at times, if something may go wrong with this huge, complex, high-tech stuff, and if you, the patient, will chiefly pay the price.

I was surprised by how quickly I became used to it all; and confident in the accuracy and control of what was being managed by the staff. As the reader will see, in the end, when I was graduating (strong habits being what they are), I missed the place; missed the very sounds, and the gigantism. Which is not surprising inasmuch as I had great faith in Dr. North and his program for me.

I was glad I had avoided a prostatectomy and equally glad I had declined watchful waiting. The latter felt too passive for my case, even though it could be argued it was the right modality for me because of my advanced age, seventy-eight. For whatever reason, and possibly physiological age had something to do with it, I needed to feel I was engaging my disease in a mortal

71

combat. Thinking back to that time as I write this, it seems mythical, like a magical scene out of *The Odyssey*.

In the treatment room today were Joy Engelson and the two Maries, Izant and Whiteson. I asked Joy Engelson how many patients the treatment room handles daily. "About forty," she said. I forgot to ask how many are prostate patients. I addressed the ladies correctly by name. Lying on the table, I asked Marie Whiteson to show me what she uses to strap my feet together. Holding up a bungee cord, she said, "We used to use tape. A patient brought this in about a year ago and we still use it."

There was a lilt in my step as I walked to the garage. I like the ladies, and I think they like me.

In the evening there was a party in a Chinese restaurant for granddaughter Annie's imminent fourth birthday. Annie behaved beautifully, and was particularly lovely to look at. Some day, hopefully (who knows what our mortality may bring?), she'll read this narrative and realize how healing her existence was for me—its beauty, agility, muscularity, sprightliness, intelligence, love of laughter, love of our private outings together; and so on. During the party she took my mind completely off my cancer. It was not until later in the evening, when a friend called to say she had heard that a mutual friend, with whom I had been out of touch for a year or two, had died of prostate cancer about a month ago, that I had a sobering reminder: my prostate cancer could kill me.

APRIL 15. Treatment 4 of 38. It was a darky day, as Susy used to say when she was a child. Dark, humid and oppressive, the kind that makes you want to hibernate. I didn't feel like bestirring myself for the radiation therapy, but I didn't have the luxury of not going.

A fiercely brooding, pretty woman in her forties sat hunched over in the waiting room, legs crossed, staring at the

They gave me pills. I'm not a pill taker, but if I have real trouble I'll take one. They said it will turn my urine orange."

"Any nausea?"

"No."

"Diarrhea?"

"No. Just pressure. Diarrhea comes later."

"Well, have a good weekend."

"You too."

Beginning to have some radiation side effects myself, I tried to rest for a marathon Cibachrome printing session tomorrow. The side effects worried me in general; and in particular because I had promised to go to Boulder. I had always been healthy and vigorous. I had been hospitalized only once, to have my tonsils out when I was thirty-four or thirty-five. I had been in excellent shape when I was involved in the helicopter crash on Mount Erebus. The sudden high altitude hadn't made me ill, though I was a fortnight short of being fifty-six, and had an occupation that could accurately be called sedentary.

I was looking forward to the Boulder Antarctic workshop conference, none of whose sponsors knew I had prostate cancer. But my imminent attendance raised disturbing questions rare for me. Would I be embarrassed by attacks of diarrhea? Would I be too tired, because of the radiation, to concentrate properly? Would I have to excuse myself at inopportune times to take naps? In short, would I be a hindrance to the conference, and would I embarrass myself by being there?

I wanted badly to go. I wanted, if possible, to postpone the inevitable confrontation that comes to all of us: that old, famous continental divide. On one side: my old vigor that had let me enjoy being in Antarctica and on the Southern Ocean; on the other, my having to regard myself, for the first time in my life, even if only minimally and temporarily, as an invalid, in my case because of radiation side effects.

Meanwhile I told myself that instead of "playing" during free times in Boulder, I would rest in my hotel room; or would

75

have convivial, supportive meetings with my friend Kurt Schlesinger, who lived in Boulder, knew I had prostate cancer, and knew I was planning to go there.

To tell or not to tell the National Science Foundation about my prostate cancer? I had no objection to telling. But I wanted to avoid being looked after, being favored because of my illness. I wanted to *escape* my illness during the pleasant time of the workshop. I wanted to feel like any other old Antarctic hand. I decided to wait a while; to see what radiation side effects, if any, I would have to deal with.

APRIL 17, 1993. Annie's fourth birthday! A new life flourishes.

The Cibachrome printing session today lasted from 9:00 to 5:00. I was nervous, tired and preoccupied. Sylvia, a classmate, though ignorant of my illness, asked, "Are you all right? I'm worried about you." I thought, "You barely know me. Why should you worry about me? Anyhow, how can you tell I'm not all right?"

Her interest, or her willingness to express it, felt like a strange invasion of my privacy. On the one hand I was flattered by her attention: she was youthful, well built, and pretty. And I tended to welcome attention, because the knowledge I had cancer made me feel I had been set apart, a winner in the wrong lottery. Aging in our time and culture isn't easy. I have a good life, and, except for the cancer, I'm healthy; yet at times I feel society's suggestions that I take myself out to the ice, like a conforming Eskimo, and sit there, gazing at eternity, until I die.

On the other hand, I preferred to be private in class; to focus entirely on trying to make good Cibachrome prints for a subject still vital to me: Antarctica; and to deal, in the solitude of my mind, with whatever feelings of mourning I had regarding the latest and most vivid evidence of my mortality: cancer. Paradox, superstition, magic: in Antarctica, until the Erebus crash, I had always felt like a child in feeling I was immortal—yes, bad things *could* happen in Antarctica; I knew a great deal about how they *had* happened; but they wouldn't ever happen to *me*. I was too much in a state of grace, simply by being in Antarctica, for them to come my way.

At home I smelled and tasted the Cibachrome processor chemicals in my nose, mouth and throat for hours. Telling Joan about this, I remarked, "I wonder if the chemicals are carcinogenic." After a pause I added, "A guy with cancer shouldn't worry about carcinogenic materials." We laughed.

APRIL 19, 1993, MONDAY. Treatment 6 of 38. The schedule for the Boulder Antarctic workshop conference arrived today. I saw that it would give me no time to rest, and would keep me away from the Boulder hotel almost entirely except for sleep time, so I began thinking it won't be good for me to attend. I regret having spent time and energy on the matter.

I met with Dr. North as scheduled this afternoon. (I'm to meet with him each Monday after my therapy, at which time I can ask questions and report any side effects.) I admire his intelligence, openness, responsiveness, and his readiness to answer or try to answer any of my questions.

"Am I being irradiated beyond the borders of my prostate?" I asked.

"Yes. It's a safety measure to ensure against some of the cancer cells having traveled beyond the gland. If you had a Gleason 5 I wouldn't need to do a standard field. But with a Gleason 6, which you have, there's a 15 percent chance of the surrounding tissues being affected. I may do a body cast for you later, when I do a conedown."

"Conedown?"

Using hand gestures suggesting a cone, he said, "In a conedown field, the standard field is reduced to a size more closely approximating the size of the prostate."

"What did you find when you did the digital?"

He had me feel the bunched muscle between his thumb and forefinger. "That's about the consistency of a normal gland," he said. He had me feel his knuckle. "That's about the way a tumor feels."

"Am I correct in thinking the anterior side of the gland isn't available in a digital exam?" I asked.

"Yes. Unfortunately, some 10 percent of prostate tumors arise on that side, and they often spread. However, the ultrasound can see the anterior side."

"What causes one person to have greater side effects than another?"

"Field size [the size of the area being irradiated]. Dosage. Monitor units. Degree of awareness."

"Does my greater than usual awareness of what's going on, due to the nature of my job in keeping a cancer journal, increase the likelihood of my having side effects?"

"Yes."

"Does radiation elevate PSA?"

"Sometimes. I won't take your PSA until a month after you finish therapy."

"I've made a guess at the length of my exposure. About nine seconds for anterior and posterior, and ten for lateral."

He smiled. "That's pretty close. But instead of time, I think of the exposure in terms of monitor units. You get 52 units respectively for front and back, and 62 respectively for the two lateral exposures."

"My stage of prostate cancer is B1?"

"Yes. Your tumor is limited to one lobe."

"What's Cerrobend, and why do we use it?"

"It's an alloy of lead, cadmium, bismuth, and possibly some other metals. We use it because of its low melting point, which makes it easy to handle in-house. Lead has a melting point of about 625° Fahrenheit. Cerrobend's melting point is only 160° Fahrenheit. You can put your finger in it when it's molten. Your finger will burn, but the tissue won't be destroyed."

"I gather I'm on closed-circuit TV during my therapy."

"Correct. Does it burn when you urinate?"

"It feels more like the head of my penis is being pinched by an instrument."

"That doesn't sound like radiation cystitis. More like a spasm in the sphincter."

APRIL 20. Treatment 7 of 38. I resigned from the Boulder conference today and canceled flight and hotel reservations. I'm relieved I'm not going to attend. But I'm disappointed I won't see my friend Kurt Schlesinger, who lives in Boulder and who was a close colleague of mine for a year at the Center for Advanced Study in the Behavioral Sciences at Stanford, 1978–79. I went to the Center soon after my third Antarctic trip, and wrote much of *Beyond Cape Horn* there. I was an anomaly there, for I'm no behavioral scientist, and no academic. I guess I was asked to come because I was planning to write an Antarctic book.

Cousin Erik reports that when Cousin Murray and his wife, Jan, visited him and Molly yesterday, Murray asked to see Erik's vacuum device for achieving an erection. (More about this device later.) Murray said his impotence is "intermittent" when he and Jan are in Florida. Erik told me that when Jan saw the device she said, "Feh! I've had enough sex in my life!"

Erik and I had quite a number of belly laughs about all this. Why are sexual problems so often the butt of jokes? Maybe, in the case of Murray and Jan, because these two nice, upstanding people are so upstandingly straight. I doubt that Jan really meant it when she said she's had enough of sex. What she probably meant was that Murray's impotence isn't going to affect her love of him; and that sex isn't so important, in their older age, that she and Murray need to embrace a vacuum device for their happiness.

This afternoon Joy Engelson handed me an appointment card for a second simulation next Monday, explaining that smaller blocks will be made while I continue therapy; thus I won't have to interrupt therapy while waiting for them. I recalled the bitter pain of catheterization. As she was spreading a fresh sheet on the patient's table, I remarked that the table is comfortable despite its surface that suggests a tennis racquet. "Most of our patients complain about the table," she said. "They say it hurts. Thin people say it hurts their back."

I fell asleep on the table today. At the conclusion of my treatment, golden-haired Marie Izant handed me a slip obliging me to get a CBC (complete blood count) at the hospital today or tomorrow. She said I'll be getting one once a week during my therapy, the purpose being to see if the radiation is causing too precipitous a drop in my counts, especially the white ones (which fight infection) and the platelets (which help prevent bleeding). "High-energy radiation can depress your immune system," she explained.

APRIL 21. Treatment 8 of 38. I felt good today; the Boulder pressure is off!

The brooding, pretty woman was in the Oncology Center waiting room this afternoon, staring as usual at the floor, head bent low, eyes shielded by large gold-rimmed glasses. She wore a flowing, deep-blue dressing gown and was hugging herself as if to keep out X rays. Her blonde hair, probably tinted, wasn't long as I had believed, but cut mannishly, with not a single hair out of place. Gray stirrup tights; black loafers; gold ear pendants; gold bracelets; gold rings. What is she being treated for?

After my treatment I went to the radiology section of the hospital; had blood drawn for my complete blood count; borrowed my bone scan and CAT scan pictures from radiology, and studied them in the viewing room, with its large light screens. I couldn't understand them, but I needed to get at least an aesthetic sense of them. I stared blankly at the 103 small CAT scan pictures. The 15 bone scan pictures (on four plates), small and very grainy, brought to mind black-and-white lithographs. My skull shots reminded me of shrunken Amazon Indian heads.

APRIL 22. Treatment 9 of 38. It's rainy and dark, and I'm unusually aware of side effects; also of general aches and pains, those gifts of old age. It seems strange to me that I can authentically describe myself as being very old.

It's becoming increasingly difficult for me to pee. Last night I was up seven or eight times. Hard to get started, hard to stop. I feel as if the head of my penis is being squeezed. And the rectal area is becoming more sensitive. At times I receive a false signal that I need to move my bowels, or that my rectal sphincter is about to relax in an embarrassing way. Toward the end of last week I felt as if I had a bad sunburn. I was flushed at times, and my skin felt crawly. I felt chilled, fluey. It tries my limited patience.

Yesterday I felt surprisingly good. Was it due to the weather? To the fact that I took Advil and vitamins the previous day? That I resigned from the Antarctic workshop, freeing myself of a degree of responsibility?

As I approached the Oncology Center waiting room this afternoon I saw that the brooding blonde woman was seated as usual in the chair with its back to the door. Nurse Debby Kuban sat opposite her. They were speaking privately. I sat down facing the door, being careful to cross my legs, for though I wore two gowns it would have been easy for someone across from me to see my naked groin. The lady wore yesterday's blue dressing gown, and now white stockings and white athletic shoes.

"Yes, I'm definitely going to call my therapist this evening," she said, rising from her chair.

She and Debby Kuban left the room. Soon afterwards Dr. North appeared in the doorway, pointed at me, and said, "May I see you for a minute," and led the way into the adjacent exam room. "I understand you had an interaction with a patient," he said.

I stared at him. "I've had no interaction."

"One of the technicians said you were upset by a woman patient."

"Not through an interaction. I remarked that I'm saddened by her sadness. I've rarely seen such sadness. It fills the waiting room. I asked no questions about her."

"I can tell you that her cancer is very curable."

"I'm glad to hear it."

"Without breaking confidentiality, I can tell you she feels that never in her life has her privacy been so invaded as it is here."

"I'm sorry for her. As you know, I feel very differently about coming here."

I mentioned that at times I have some burning in the tip of my penis when I urinate.

"Are you about to burst with the need to pee when you come here?" he asked.

"No. I take a leak just before leaving the house. I drink a large cup and a half of water."

"That's not enough. You're coming with an empty bladder. It won't harm you if you have therapy once or twice with an empty bladder, but you'll increase the side effects if you fail to come with a full one."

"I thought the water I drink just before leaving the house is sufficient to distend the bladder by the time I have my treatment."

"Try not to pee for two hours before your therapy."

We parted soon afterwards, but not before I learned with relief that he doesn't plan to catheterize me or to insert a rectal probe for the new simulation on Monday. He said they're not necessary this time.

APRIL 23, 1993. Treatment 10 of 38. I've finished my second week of therapy!

Sylvia, of my Cibachrome class, called this afternoon. "I'm worried about you," she said. "I sense you're going through something."

"It's sweet of you to worry about me, but I'm okay," I said.

What does she know? And from whom? I'm not keeping my cancer a secret, but I'd rather not have it known in class. I don't care to run into it (and myself) every time I go there. Also, she's only thirty and no doubt has her own problems, and I'd rather spare her such knowledge.

APRIL 24, 1993. My Cibachrome session today lasted from 9:00 to 2:15, during which time I never sat down. I had pains in the groin and rectal areas from being on my feet so long. The pains made me tired and jumpy. Joan said it sounds like a woman having her period. I need a day of rest to let the radiation side effects subside.

Six

April 26 to May 16, 1993

Because I had a potentially fatal disease, and because of the possibility that my radiotherapy might bring unpleasant and even serious side effects, I was intensely curious about how things worked in this domain. I wanted to confront and absorb relevant knowledge, as a consequence of which questions often seemed to rise spontaneously in my mind. No doubt my motivation was partly, and possibly largely, due to Dr. North's enthusiasm regarding his specialty, which he readily communicated to me, and to his willingness, even eagerness, to help me understand the various goings-on.

At the very outset of our relationship I sensed a great care in him about the health of my curiosity, almost as if he were my psychotherapist as well as my radiation oncologist, and I became acutely aware of how lucky I was to have encountered such a kindly, empathetic and intelligent doctor, in whom I had so much trust. I looked forward to our meetings, with their frequent question-and-answer sessions, because of the intellectual pleasure they gave me and because I was convinced that his interaction with me was profoundly and positively affecting my radiotherapy.

But this, of course, didn't mean I took it for granted I'd be cured. As we all know, cancer has a wisdom, a power, a sovereignty of its own, and its concern for us humans is about as real as that of Antarctica, with its great mountain ranges, fabulous light, and unearthly cold.

APRIL 26, 1993, MONDAY. Treatment 11 of 38. Meeting with Dr. North in an exam room this afternoon, I asked a question that had been on my mind the past week. "Why haven't the benign prostate cells learned to travel, whereas the cancer prostate cells love to take trips?"

Tall, dark-bearded, he smiled. "If you could answer that, you'd win a Nobel Prize," he replied. "There are a number of theories. The one I subscribe to is this. During embryological development, human cells replicate rapidly and can travel almost anywhere. For example, you may find testicle cells in the abdomen. That's the nature of human cells at that time. At a certain stage of development a protein adheres to the DNA. Its function is to restrict replication and travel. Without it we'd never develop into complete human beings. Apparently, with age the effect of the protein on the DNA diminishes, so some of the prostate cells 'regress' to the embryological stage, and they replicate and travel."

"So is it a case of old age being not simply a second childhood, as folklore has it, but a second fetus-state?"

"In a sense, yes. If the theory is correct. Let's go to the sim [simulation] room and do your conedown simulation."

We went to the room, on the right of the treatment room, in which I had had my first simulation.

"See those lasers?" he said. "We're going to set them up so that, although we can't see them, they're going to be intersecting in your prostate gland. However, I don't mean they'll actually penetrate your body, the way the X rays will. Also, we're going to be making a body cast for you, which consists of a bunch of chemicals we'll mix together in that large silver plastic bag over there. The bag will go on the table, and you'll lie on it, and the chemicals will grow up around you while becoming quite warm, and will turn hard. This will form the cast.

The cast will make it possible for you to lie almost exactly in the same position each time you have a treatment. In the cone-down mode we'll be aiming at a smaller field, so greater pin-point accuracy will be required. After we make the cast, we'll take pictures. I don't need to catheterize you, because I already did that for your first simulation. I already know precisely where your bladder and rectum are."

Cybill, a technician, poured the chemicals into the sack and placed the sack on the gurney. I lay on the gurney, my hips on the sack. Cybill bound my feet with tape. Heat of the chemicals. Hot tailbone. Hot left testicle. As a favor to me, Dr. North filmed me with a camcorder so I would later be able, if necessary, to describe the scene.

"Although you're a writer, I still think that one picture is worth more than a thousand words," he said teasingly. I laughed. "You might disagree with me."

I'm not ordinarily used to being very passive, as I had to be in radiotherapy. His comment therefore surprised as well as pleased me, bringing me, as it did, out of a kind of half-sleep.

"Well, pictures are not as good at depicting psychological or emotional events," I said from my patient's cocoon state.

"Right. Although they can stir emotions."

Four simulation pictures of me were taken with weaker X rays than those that would be used in my radiotherapy. Then Cybill shot me with a Polaroid camera so the technicians would be able to see how I had been oriented on the table.

As I left the Oncology Center I spotted an old friend and neighbor leaving the Medical Center. We greeted each other with smiles. Nodding toward the building behind me, she asked suspiciously, "What were you doing in there?"

"I have prostate cancer."

She gave me a long, sad, empathetic stare. "I'm sorry!" she cried, and hugged me.

"No big deal," I said as we walked toward the garage.

"I've just had a mammogram. Tell me about your cancer."

"I'm getting radiation. I've had two weeks of it. Five and a half to go. An expensive way to get a laxative."

"Oh? I never heard that."

"It's par for the course."

This evening I learned that Cousin Murray's PSA after radiation is only 0.5. How wonderful!

APRIL 28. Treatment 13 of 38. I'm feeling radiation side effects sooner than I expected. I'm cold all the time, I need lots of sleep, and my groin feels extremely vulnerable. No walk or writing today. I'm too tired.

In order to attend the support group meeting this afternoon, I had rescheduled my therapy for 12:45 (normally it was at 2:15); therefore I needed to be especially aware of when I could last pee before going for my treatment. I decided that my last pee should be at 10:40; and I urinated at that time. Then I made a serious error by drinking two or three large cups of water afterwards. Not surprisingly, by the time I found a parking spot in the garage, I already needed to void.

As I sat in the Oncology Center waiting room, nervously glancing at my watch, I urgently had to go, and I doubted my ability to hold it in. I wanted to tell nurse Debby Kuban, who was standing in front of the high nurses' counter, about my problem, but she was busily talking with a tall man in a hospital gown. The only other person in the waiting room was a fully dressed older man, whose appointment preceded mine. The man pointed at his nose (there was a bump there, the middle of which was much darker than flesh), and explained he was being treated for cancer.

Finally, when Debby was free, I went over and spoke to her, my legs trembling with my need to urinate. "Go!" she said sympathetically, touching my shoulder.

"But Dr. North is concerned about my being irradiated on an empty bladder."

She strode to the waiting room doorway, glanced in, asked the man which doctor he was waiting to see, and turned to me and said, "You're next! They'll be ready in a minute or two!"

The Marie with the golden hair (Izant) motioned for me to follow her to the treatment room. "I saw you dancing," she said when I was lying on the table. "You mustn't hold it in so long."

"But I need to have my bladder distended so it avoids the field. How embarrassing!"

"Why? I dance myself sometimes. The X-ray bathroom is being repaired, so people come to use ours, and sometimes it's full."

She and the other Marie (Whiteson), who also was aware of my problem, worked fast to help me. My bladder pressure had become alarmingly great. The huge machine was directly above me, and I was extremely aware of each zap. Normally I would recoil a bit inwardly at the buzzing that accompanied each shot, but now I was eager to hear it, and immeasurably eager to have today's treatment over with.

By the time there was only one shot left, the head of my penis felt ready to explode, and my bladder ached frighteningly. I was horrified—was I about to leak several drops onto the table? Should I ask Marie Izant to stop the machine?

I squeezed my urinary sphincter as hard as I could. "Idiot!" it cried, "I'm exhausted! I hate you! I'm going to let go!" "Please don't!" I begged.

The session finally ended, and I quickly said my good-byes, crying, "Never again!" as I hurried to the dressing room bathroom, where my sphincter was so stunned I had trouble starting. At last, slowly, the flow came, and slowly the pains subsided.

I got dressed; made my way to the hospital registration section; received authorization for my complete blood count; went to the radiology waiting room; took a seat; and waited for my turn to have blood drawn.

My friend John Lowrance called at about 9:00 P.M. "How're you doing?" he asked.

"The radiation takes only seconds, yet this evening I feel like a zombie."

"You're getting strong medicine."

"Let me tell you a joke I heard today at the support group. Why do some urologists use two fingers to do a rectal digital exam?"

Long pause. "Why?"

"To get a second opinion."

He slowly cracked up.

APRIL 29, 1993. Treatment 14 of 38. Today I avoided pee torture by peeing as late as 1:30 before drinking one and a half cups of water.

At the beginning of therapy, as I was being adjusted on the table (at times there's a tiny tugging at my legs or feet or shoulders or thighs; I'm not allowed to help), I asked Christina Dimaggio, who has short brown hair and limpid gray eyes, when I'll start using the conedown blocks. She checked in a looseleaf book and reported, "As of today you've had fourteen days of standard blocks. You'll stay on them for twenty-five days, then go to the smaller, conedown ones."

Toward the end of the session I asked golden-haired Marie to outline with a marker the front and side areas of my body that were being irradiated; I wanted to be able to see how large the fields were. She readily complied. I sensed from the pressure of the marker on my hips that the fields are much larger than I had imagined. When she drew my abdominal/pelvic field I was startled, for she went down to just above the base of my penis. I immediately recalled the possibility of becoming impotent because of radiation therapy.

As I left the table Christina asked, "Would you like to see a couple of pictures of your fields?"

She had stuck them on a light screen. They were enlarged pictures of my pelvic area. One was a frontal view, another a lateral one. They contained in brown marker my standard fields,

90

and in blue my conedown fields. The conedown were significantly smaller than the standard ones.

"See the balloon in your bladder?" she asked, pointing to a little round spot. "It helped locate the place in your bladder."

I hadn't realized a balloon had been inserted with the catheter during my first simulation. She pointed out my bowel and rectum. My pelvis was sharply delineated, but it was unclear to me where my prostate was. I was startled to see how far down the brown (standard-field) line went.

"My whole pubic area is being irradiated," I thought. "No wonder impotence may sometimes result."

Back in the dressing room at the end of my treatment, I was almost finished dressing, when there was a knock on the door.

"Come in," I said.

It was Dr. North. "Mr. Neider, I understand you had a rough time with urination yesterday."

"I almost didn't make it."

"Change that by an hour. Take your last leak at 1:00 instead of 12:00. I don't want you to be that uncomfortable."

"Good. By the way, is it correct that radiation therapy can't be given more than once?"

"Yes. We give the tissues about as much as they can handle. They remember what they got. Give them more and you may slough out the bladder and rectum."

My body is unpredictable these days. Today I felt good, and put the feeling to good use: I worked hard at writing most of the day.

APRIL 30, 2:40 P.M. Treatment 15 of 38. My heart, lungs and digestive system are crying, "Don't you see how unhappy we are? We need exercise! So why aren't you walking?"

"I'm too tired. Try to be patient," I reply.

"Why are you letting them do this to us?"

"Don't you understand it can't be helped?"

My bladder and urinary sphincter are hurting. "Why are you torturing us?" they ask.

"I'm trying to make the best of a rough situation," I explain. "To use a vulgar but accurate expression, the radiation is knocking the shit out of me."

My upper stomach cries, "Don't you see that your not walking is giving me indigestion? You've eaten rich stuff. You need to walk it off!"

"I'm just as addicted to walking as you are," I counter. "But I'm too tired. Think of it this way: we must all give up something for the general good, otherwise the whole system will collapse."

When I told Cousin Erik about the low-residue diet suggested for me because of my radiation (eggnog, ice cream, and other foods rich in cholesterol), he remarked, "They try to kill you one way or another."

At times I think, "Why did I eat too much at dinner? What's driving me? Who's rocking the boat?"

I'm having to adjust to a new identity. I half-feel I'm on another planet, looking down at the human drama as if it's spread out like the peasants in a Breughel painting.

8:15 P.M. I'm tired down into my bones. The usual aches and pains are magnified. Burning sensation all day in the "trigger point" in the left side of my nape.

MAY 1, 1993. A dream last night.

My daughter and I are at a farm. There are large rooms with lots of animals, including large exotic hens. An aggressive hen pecks at my fly, grabs hold of it. I'm startled. I clutch her by the neck, squeeze hard, feel her neck beginning to creak. She lets go. Moments later I see her aggressively fighting with a young horse. I shout, "Susy, look! The hen and horse are fighting!" The horse's long neck lunges. Its jaws grab the hen's head, start crunching it.

Awaking, I sense a connection between the dream and the threat to my potency inherent in the X-ray field's coming down as far as the base of my penis.

I had a full walk today. It was sunny, 80 degrees in the afternoon, but until I got in the stride of my power walk I was strangely chilly, as if from a bad sunburn.

"Think of the good side," I reminded myself. "If you had chosen surgery you'd be healing a large wound. And would be incontinent, busy with diapers. And probably impotent. And you'd be unable to do your power walks. You can walk, you can print Cibachrome, you can write. So quit complaining."

But, focusing on my present discomfort, I tended to forget how lucky I am the cancer didn't spread, and that I had the option of selecting radiation as against surgery.

I turned in early and slept deeply, but was interrupted seven or eight times by an urgent need to pee, which produced little volume for the effort.

"I want to pee!" cried my bladder. "I want to go too!" immediately shouted my bowel, determined not to be outshone. Usually my bowel's cry is a false alarm. And my bladder's is partly false inasmuch as a poor stream results.

At one point I found myself thinking, "Don't bug me, bowel! You're a pain in the ass!" But why shouldn't these citizens of my body politic make their needs known? The benign tissues (and presumably both bladder and bowel are benign) are innocent bystanders of an "ethnic cleansing" going on. "Out, out, damned spots!" cry the X rays in their savage healing work. The rays fight fire with invisible fire.

My body had been running along with relative smoothness for generations. True, it had had its share of charley horses and other muscle and tendon pains, as well as an occasional mild illness; but for the most part the interior parts, the organs, had been functioning silently, had been well oiled, quiescent, doing their job without much consultation with doctors and me. Now they seemed to have become aborigines, seemed even to be deranged, and threatening to make their private condition public; or had already done so, as far as I was concerned. Furthermore, they were not so much consulting with me as demanding: do this, that and the other! or we'll burn your house down, or perform other, more personal, acts of violence. I had a sense, at times, that I, or what was left of me, extraordinarily law-abiding and mild-mannered, was being confronted by a bunch of *yakuza* (Japanese mafia types).

On another level, I was aware that radiation in the pelvic area sometimes exacts a considerable price: for example, ulceration of the tip of the bladder, or of the rectum; or causes long-lasting and possibly permanent proctitis (inflammation and bleeding of the rectum); or worse, can so injure the rectum as to require corrective surgery and, for a time, a colostomy to allow the rectum to heal. (A colostomy is an incision in the abdominal wall and colon to create an artificial anus.) In short, my occasional anxiety wasn't entirely due to an active imagination.

However, current radiotherapy is a great advance over the practice of twenty or thirty years ago, and while I note these facts for the record, and because they were a true part of my state of mind, I also urge the reader to be firmly aware that the chance of having severe side effects has greatly decreased.

When, in July 1993, a month after my radiotherapy was completed, and Dr. North, at my request, had read an early draft of the present narrative, he said he felt let down by my not having informed him about my intense side effects. "I could have spared you at least some of them," he said emotionally. "There were things I could have prescribed. Why didn't you tell me? I had no idea you were suffering as much as you were. I checked back through my notes, and there was nothing about such side effects!"

I felt very bad. I hadn't meant to keep him in the dark. I had simply assumed that, whereas in some patients there were few or no side effects, in others there were many; and that these many were as "normal" as the lack of side effects. I assumed that mine were partly caused by my awareness of what was happening; a necessary awareness because of the nature of the journal I was keeping; a journal that increasingly led me to think a potential book was involved.

I did my best to explain what had happened. I felt sheepish nevertheless. On the other hand, as we both knew, all drugs have some side effects, and possibly I would have reacted poorly to the prescribed drugs.

When I mentioned his reaction to Joan, she said, "Didn't you once tell me you didn't want to disguise any side effects? And I said, 'Oh, so you don't want to disguise them! In that case, don't you dare gripe!' Maybe you took my prohibition against griping too seriously."

I related her remarks to Dr. North, and we both had a good laugh, and that was the end of the "let down" episode.

MAY 3, 1993. Treatment 16 of 38. When I met with Dr. North in the usual exam room after my therapy today, I told him about my bad anal burning, so he examined my anus briefly to check the degree of irritation. We're engaged in a partnership; we have a goal in common and are not obsessed with niceties. He prescribed suppositories and a salve, both of which contain hydrocortisone.

"Are my side effects on schedule?" I asked.

"Your body has read the literature and is following side effect instructions to the letter. You're on the curve."

I told him how, sometimes, when my bladder says it wants to urinate, my bowel cries it wants out too.

"That's right," he commented. "When the bowel surrounds feces, it feels swollen, and this swelling tells the brain to order it to eliminate. The bowel wall is currently swollen from radiation. The bowel isn't bright, it confuses the two kinds of swelling, so it asks the brain to order an elimination, and manages to confuse the brain too, partly."

"How long will it be after therapy is completed before my side effects disappear?"

"In about two weeks after therapy you should feel a good deal better. Normally a patient recovers fully in about a month."

"Would it be possible to do a TURP [transurethral resection of the prostate] after therapy?"

"Yes, but cautiously, and by a skillful urologist. There *is* a chance of scar tissue forming and blocking the urethra, necessitating a reaming operation."

MAY 5, 1993. Treatment 18 of 38. Yesterday I felt fine. I worked well, and probably too long. And I stayed up too late. In short, I overdid it, and today am paying the price. Also, yesterday was bright. Today is dark, gloomy. I feel jumpy, restless, ill. Some days on going to therapy I feel warm-bodied and confident. At others, like today, I feel an extra sense of vulnerability, as if I'm coming down with the flu.

I'm eating too much, probably to relax, so I often have heartburn. And I'm taking too seriously something I read somewhere: that you shouldn't lose weight during therapy.

This morning I felt discomfort in the perineal region, as in prostatitis, and pain at the beginning and end of urination. And last night I kept getting up to pee and tried not to get angry about it. It's easy these days for me to get angry at my body.

Recently I've often felt like an invalid. The radiation, piercing my hips, has affected my gait. I especially notice this when walking from the garage to the Oncology Center. Is it obvious to others?

I rarely flinch when the buzzing of the X-ray machine starts, though I know I'm about to be roasted internally. Whenever I have a negative image such as roasting, I remind myself that the machine is designed to save my life, or at least to prolong it.

Tomorrow is the halfway point in my therapy. On the one hand I'm pleased, on the other I groan inwardly when I think how much more I have to go. Nancy Stevenson, a receptionist, remarked today, "My goodness! You've already had three weeks? How time flies! The rest will whiz by!" But for me time drags its heels.

Despite feeling like an invalid, I left the house at 4:45 today for Mercer County Community College to beat the traffic; worked on photo notes there until 6:00; began printing Antarctic slides on 11 × 14 Cibachrome paper (really polyester); and worked without stopping until 9:30. It was painful to stand; my groin and rectum hurt; but I was astonished by my success this evening: four good prints in four tries! Joan said they're admirable, which greatly pleased me.

MAY 7, 1993, FRIDAY. Treatment 20 of 38. Yesterday was lovely, but I was too tired to walk after therapy. My therapy can accurately be described as a pain in the ass, both literally and figuratively. It's hard to concentrate on my work when parts of my body, out of synch, are urgently making me aware of them. My rectum and anus keep threatening to have a movement. Reluctantly I go to the bathroom. False alarm. I'm getting tired of being threatened in this way. But sometimes the threats are real. At least I don't have diarrhea—yet.

A friend called to say she's sorry I have prostate cancer, and that her husband also had had it, and was treated last February with cryosurgery (destruction of the prostate by freezing). Before surgery his PSA was 13. It was this number that had caused his urologist to suspect he had cancer. After surgery it was a startling 0.07.

I took my usual walk today (the first in a week), and felt almost sick afterwards. Strange week: I felt so good on Tuesday, almost normal, then went downhill day after day.

MAY 10, 1993. Treatment 21 of 38. Dr. North, tall, straight, youthful, dark-bearded, smiling, appeared in the doorway of the waiting room and motioned for me to enter one of the exam rooms.

"I have some questions to ask," I said in the room. He nodded. "Why irradiate the bowel and bladder?"

"We could more specifically irradiate your prostate through the lateral fields; that is, through your hips. But we'd damage the hip bones. You'd get severe arthritis. So we spread the radiation by also doing the front and back, and thereby preserve the hips."

"What do you call side effects that are permanent?"

"Late tissue reaction."

"Is there a correlation between prostate cancer and sperm count?"

"No."

"Between prostate cancer and production of testosterone?"

"We're not sure. But we know that testosterone stimulates the cancer, which is why the testicles are removed if the cancer has spread; or why hormone therapy is used."

"Is there a correlation between prostate cancer and benign prostatic hypertrophy [enlargement]?"

"No."

"Do eunuchs develop prostate cancer in old age?"

He smiled. "I would doubt it."

"Will therapy shrink my gland?"

"Maybe a little. Including the benign part."

"What about John Darrough, whom you'll meet at the support group when you address it on the 26th? He had radiation six years ago and his prostate cancer has recurred. It's limited to the gland. His PSA is 18, I think. What can be done for him?"

"They'll probably watch it. If it spreads, they may give him hormone therapy. Or chemotherapy."

"So in his case radiation wasn't a cure. I wonder why not."

"I don't know. We'd need to know the specifics. The kind of treatment he received. How aggressive it was."

"Are the irradiated areas likely to become scar tissue some years down the road? You remember I mentioned I had a massive dose of X rays at Columbia-Presbyterian for a plantar wart many years ago, and that fourteen years later I had scar tissue at the site."

"Some scarring probably will occur to replace the space left by the dead cancer cells."

"Was a little balloon attached to the catheter during my simulation?"

"Yes."

"To hold the catheter in place?"

"Yes. Also, I put some dye in the balloon to make it more opaque so I could see exactly where we were."

"Will the conedown fields still use 180 rads?"

"Yes."

"How does the amount of radiation I receive compare with that of a nuclear accident like Chernobyl?"

"The human body tolerates radiation in a small area much better than across the whole body. If you exposed a hundred people to the amount of radiation *you* receive in two days—exposed their whole bodies—about half would die."

"Is it true a prostate cancer cure is a cure only because you'll die before the cancer gets you?"

"Absolutely not. I'm going to try to kill every prostate cancer cell in your body. If you live fifty years longer, you won't have prostate cancer."

"So how am I doing?"

"Very well.

MAY 11, 1993. Treatment 22 of 38. This morning I chatted by phone with Walter Abelson, 71, the man who had cryosurgery. Last July while on Martha's Vineyard, having urinary problems, he thought he was experiencing another kidney stone, but a check at the local emergency room was negative. When he returned to New York and saw his urologist he learned his PSA was elevated. A second PSA was also high: 13.

In September he had an ultrasound biopsy that indicated he had cancer in one lobe. He doesn't know his Gleason score. A bone scan and CAT scan showed the cancer hadn't spread. His urologist said his cancer was curable by any one of three methods.

(1) Prostatectomy. His urologist advised against this as being too invasive and having too many side effects.

(2) Radiation therapy. His urologist was hesitant about this because it can't be repeated.

(3) Cryosurgery, which his urologist recommended because about three years ago it began producing some good results, and because it can be repeated. Also, a doctor who was performing the operation was a friend of the urologist.

Abelson's operation, involving a spinal and an ultrasound, and performed through the rectal wall, took a couple of hours, after which, regaining consciousness, he was taken to the recovery room. He was not allowed to leave the room until he could feel sensation in his toes some six hours later. Meanwhile his wife anxiously paced a hospital corridor.

When he left the hospital he was still wearing a suprapubic tube (between navel and penis) for peeing. He wore the tube and Kotex for about four weeks. The tube had a cap he could screw off. For a while, when he used the tube, there was some blood in his urine. He could also urinate naturally, but this at first produced only a small volume.

When the tube was removed, the suprapubic opening was stitched up. He had no incontinence; but he did become impotent. It's uncertain how long it will take before he regains his potency, if ever. For a while he had a problem with fatigue and had to nap daily around noon. After a time, resuming his jogging schedule, he discovered he no longer needed to nap. As of today his penis "still feels numb and sensitive."

I get up early, feeling great. I'm in harmony with the weather and people. My step is jaunty, my muscles feel oiled. It's a pleasure to bend over and lift things. What's causing this change? A week ago, on another Tuesday, I also felt great. Why? I sense it's important to know, so I can take steps to feel like this more often.

"Don't change a thing," I advise myself. "Hang on to this mood, this condition, whatever it is."

By noon, suddenly exhausted, I'm obliged to sit in the lounger and shut my eyes. Aching down into my bones, I absolutely must drift off for at least fifteen minutes. "The nap will give me a second burst of energy," I think. Wrong. The crash, like a stealth bomber, comes without warning. Even as I sit in the lounger, giving way to rest, I'm not allowed to be restful. My bowel keeps threatening to have a third (or a fourth?) movement.

"Give me a *break*," I think. Or I think slyly, "Maybe if I pee, the bowel will leave me alone." Sometimes this strategy works.

My body, under assault, understandably is counterattacking. But how can I think sanely in this state? Last night I awoke nine or ten times to pee urgently, painfully—in ridiculously short bursts that angered me. "Anger will only keep you awake and make the morning even stranger than it's already likely to be," I told myself.

I'd like to visit Cousin Erik this weekend, my first without a Saturday Cibachrome class. I haven't visited him and his wife, Molly, in weeks. But how can I do it? The drive is long, tiring. Yet that's not the chief problem. If I'm going to have a night of strange peeing or a day of unexpected bowel movements, I'll be much better off at home. Also, when the fatigue hits, it makes me unsociable.

Last Sunday, when Susy, Whitney, and Annie came over for Mother's Day, it was wonderful to see them, but when I sat in the lounger watching Annie cavort (her four-year-old body has muscular needs), each of her sudden, broad movements and any loud sound caused me pain. And the great spray of white lilacs Susy brought Joan were lovely to look at. Ordinarily I love lilacs ("When lilacs last in the dooryard bloomed. . . ."), but now their odor seemed bitter, strong, pungent. Of course, I said nothing. Mustn't spoil healthy people's fun.

Parts of my body, especially the bowel and bladder, are angry. They're irritated, inflamed, swollen, and are blaming me for their condition. They make sudden demands. I go downstairs in the morning to make a coffee. Suddenly, urgently, I must move my bowels. I abruptly stop what I'm doing.

"Go screw yourself!" I say to my bowel. Then, realizing what I'm saying (and feeling), I change my tune. "I know you're having a hard time," I say, "and that it's not your fault, that you're doing the best you can. I'm sorry for you. But what can I do?"

I'm dealing with rebellions. How can I concentrate when my body makes such demands?

MAY 14, 1993, FRIDAY. Treatment 25 of 38. This is my worst day since beginning therapy. My body complains bitterly all over. I'm beginning to suspect I'm suffering from walk deprivation. I last walked last Sunday, five days ago, and before that I hadn't walked for a full week. I'm a walk addict, I've walked hard all my life. I think I'm having withdrawal symptoms. I'm too exhausted to walk today, but if the weather allows I'll walk tomorrow and, if necessary, do nothing but rest the remainder of the day.

When I lived in the Columbia University area of Manhattan I used to walk seven miles a day. Sometimes I'd walk fourteen. My route was from 114th Street near Broadway (later it was from 118th Street and Morningside Drive) to the George Washington Bridge and back, always using Riverside Drive. There were earlier Princeton times when I used to swim the crawl at the Y almost daily, and there was another period when I cycled twenty miles a day. Nowadays in Princeton whenever I can, which in good weather may be daily, I walk three miles in about forty-three or forty-four minutes, doing about four miles an hour.

Currently, my GI tract and bladder and bowel are in an uproar. But my heart and lungs don't care about them; they have their own needs that must be met. So do my walk muscles. It will be interesting to see how I feel after I walk tomorrow, although it may take a day or two to sense the difference.

I have extremely urgent, painful and incomplete bowel movements, which occur only in the morning and can be as much as two hours apart. The bowel shuts down abruptly and forcefully, leaving me wondering why, for I feel there's more to come. Meanwhile I feel half-nauseous and half-sick, and distracted and irritable. Sometimes the whole day is colored by these morning events and emotions, and I feel I'm creeping around like a genuine invalid. Other days I make a miraculous, smiling recovery.

As the week progresses I grow noticeably more frail, vulnerable, irritable, withdrawn. By Friday, a simple Monday or Tuesday activity, like a long walk, seems vastly beyond my strength and endurance. What's the alternative? Bed rest? I'm not sick enough for that. Instead, I nap several times, briefly but deeply. I've heard of people quitting, or threatening to quit, chemotherapy. What would happen if I quit radiation after this, my fifth week?

Glancing into a mirror, I'm greeted by a frowning old man whose face has been scarred by surgery for many instances of basal cell carcinoma, a relatively mild form of skin cancer, which rarely metastasizes. My buttocks ache. What from? Too much sitting in the lounger? My waist has expanded surprisingly; I have trouble finding lightweight trousers that still fit. I haven't put on much if any weight since beginning therapy; so is my waist swollen, or have my abdominal muscles sagged through insufficient use? It hurts to pull in my gut, which is probably why I don't do it. And I'm cold, creaky, while the rest of the world, it seems, is warm, even hot.

MAY 16, 1993, SUNDAY. There are times when I have the illusion I'm close to death, and that all I need to do is close my eyes and let go. But when I shut my eyes the result is always the same: I drop off into a profound sleep from which I awake numb and disoriented for an hour. Are these signals coming from death itself; that is, from the dying of cells? If so, should they be accompanied by minor funerary obeisances?

Yesterday I walked in the morning and rested all day, napping in the living-room lounger and reading in *Two Years Before the Mast*. I think I feel better but am not positive it's due to the walk. Maybe the full resting is what's doing it. Today I repeated yesterday's routine. I walked and napped and read, and am at greater peace with myself, not only mentally but physically. My breathing is deeper, more regular, my body more relaxed, my legs and feet less achy. I'm going to give walking a high priority next week.

Seven

May 17 to June 4, 1993

MAY 17, 1993. Treatment 26 of 38. I took it easy most of the day, resting, and reading in Richard Henry Dana's wonderful *Two Years Before the Mast*. In the treatment room my new body cast was ready on the patient's table. The lady techs had let me wear my blue gown, together with my hospital gown, during standard-field therapy, but now that we were starting to use the cone-down fields, they insisted I remove it, because it might bunch up under me and affect the precision of the machine's lineup.

Taking it off, I sat on the table and hiked myself up onto the cast. Marie Izant spread a pillowcase over my waist. I lifted my hips. She pulled my hospital gown up to my chest, and my naked groin and buttocks felt the cool air. After the four zaps, I lifted myself up and slid forward beyond the cast. In the process my pubic region was unavoidably exposed to anyone in front of me. Leaving the table, I said to Marie Izant, "With the body cast, it's hard for me to protect my modesty."

"We won't look," she said with a smile.

The whole treatment room, including the ceiling, is lead-lined. Its electrically operated lead door weighs two thousand pounds. The hinges are huge. The techs and nurses wear radiation badges, also called film badges, which monitor the amount of radiation, if any, they're exposed to. Each badge contains a little strip of special film. The techs also wear a black ring containing film.

Meeting with Dr. North briefly in one of the exam rooms, I asked, "Did you say there's a 25 percent chance of impotence?"

"Yes."

"When does impotence usually occur?"

"Six months to two years after therapy. Men who are more active sexually are less likely to become impotent. Use it or lose it."

"When does diarrhea usually start?"

"Around the end of the fourth week."

"So I'm doing pretty well?"

"Very well."

"What would happen if a person in my stage of therapy would quit?"

"He might be 'cured,' but the recurrence rate would be higher."

"Is my waist swollen? I notice my trousers are tighter, yet I haven't gained weight."

"It's not your waist. Your intestines may be a bit bloated."

"Would it have been useful to do a biopsy without ultrasound four years ago? That's when a doctor at Columbia-Presbyterian wanted to do it."

"Although it's possible you had early cancer then, it's extremely unlikely it would have been picked up without an ultrasound. And Dr. Gilroy, in treating you in the years since then, didn't find cancer."

MAY 19. Abominable weather: cold, dark, rainy. I want to huddle, hibernate. I suspect this weather aggravates my side effects, maybe because it causes my body to take on water, swelling already swollen tissues. Also, I suffer easily from light deprivation. I loved being in Antarctica, particularly in continental, high-latitude Antarctica, which knows no night in summer. Also, it probably doesn't help that I drink vodka, which is acidy.

These days I'm like a pregnant woman in craving foods I rarely indulge in: creamed herring; Nova Scotia belly lox with cream cheese; canned peaches and heavy cream. I gave up eating lots of chocolate because it brought on heartburn. But my mental outlook remains good, though at times I fear I'm losing some of my sense of humor about this healing process. No therapy today; the linear accelerator was down for preventive maintenance.

In the evening I chatted for three hours with Sylvia, a tall, married Cibachrome classmate, who said, for the second time, that she'd like to spend a day in New York with me, so I finally had to tell her about my cancer, and about my therapy ending on June 4. I said I had prostate cancer; was getting radiation for it; and had some pretty strong side effects that made it inadvisable for me to spend a day away from home; but that I'd gladly do it a couple of weeks after June 4.

As I was speaking I tried not to concentrate on her reaction, but I couldn't help noticing her surprised look, and then her attempt to suppress the look's changing to one of shock. She handled the news better than I expected, and I admired her for it. Her eyes were warm, empathetic. "She's more mature than I thought," I told myself, and was glad I liked her. But I had lost my class incognito as far as my cancer was concerned. "I'll send you prayers," she said.

MAY 20, 1993. Treatment 28 of 38. I've had 71 percent of my scheduled treatments, and the side effects are increasing markedly. So grin and bear it. This morning my body feels no benefits from yesterday's holiday. Peeing, and moving my bowels, are both painful, and I'm tired and irritable all over. Last night I must have been awakened nine or ten times to pee. After a while I had to concentrate hard to avoid getting angry. By morning I felt I was a wreck.

I've already had four bowel movements, with anal burning that takes longer and longer to subside. No diarrhea yet. Maybe I'll be spared it. I think the problem is my swollen bowel and rectum. The anal canal has been greatly narrowed, so it resists

107

elimination until the pressure is considerable, and it and the sphincter shut down before the elimination is complete. I judge this by the stringiness of the stools. Poor bowel, it doesn't know what hit it, and, to add insult to injury, I'm rarely sympathetic. I hate having my concentration interrupted.

As I lay on the therapy table today I said to Marie Izant, who was on my left, "I think I'm losing my hair."

"Where?"

"Down there."

"You are," said smiling Christina of the limpid gray eyes on my right.

"Some prostate patients expect to lose the hair on their *head*," said Marie.

I ran into Dr. North in the Oncology Center lobby. We smiled at each other. "How's your treatment going? Any side effects?" I asked, deadpan.

He grinned. "Would you like to stand in for me a day or two?" he said.

MAY 24, 1993. Treatment 30 of 38. I felt better day before yesterday, had more energy than usual currently, and I had only *one* bowel movement, praise the Lord! And yesterday I spent five hours chatting with Flora, an attractive and witty single Cibachrome classmate, at Forrestal Village outside Princeton, and I wasn't tired when we split. But this morning I paid the price (do the crime; do the time) by feeling shitty.

"Pretty exclusive club, isn't it? Toughest club in the world to get into."

Said by a tall, craggy man in the waiting room today, who reminded me of Edward Hopper, the American painter, whom I knew at the Huntington Hartford Foundation in Pacific Palisades, California, in the spring of 1957 and whom I visited later on Cape Cod. Using a straw, he drank from a high, covered, orange plastic cup. Another man was a Yul Brynner: shiny, shaved, pink and grayish bald head. He wore navy trunks under his hospital gown, and long white socks with three horizontal black bands at the top. He had a different cancer from prostate; if he had prostate cancer he wouldn't be wearing trunks. Several of his front lower teeth were missing. He had trouble speaking clearly. What was he being treated for? Edward Hopper abruptly left the room as I continued reading "The Last Cranes of Siberia" by Peter Matthiessen in *The New Yorker*.

"This is the first time I've come without a chauffeur. I'm a little nervous," confessed a large-face woman with long gray hair, who wore blue trousers under her hospital gown. What was *she* being treated for?

"It's a holy congregation today," said a very tall man huskily, studying us on entering the small room. "Why are they backed up? You been treated?" he asked me.

I nodded. This being Monday, I was waiting for Dr. North to call me for our weekly meeting.

"Anybody else?"

"No," said the shy man with the large sad eyes in the corner, who had bloated-looking, shiny skin as if from too much cortisone, and a large circular thigh bruise above his right knee.

"They tacked a couple of days onto me," said the very tall man, sitting down. "They told me I'll be finished in two weeks."

"*Four* is what they told *me*," said the man in the corner.

"*Six*," said large-face Mrs. Bluepants.

"They keep you guessing," said the very tall man, and told about how great it is at Fox/Chase in Philadelphia, and about his pill, Hytrin (terazosin). "Best to take it at night, because it makes you sleepy," he explained. "Helps about 50 percent. Usually with the pill I go just three times at night. Somebody said I might have to stay on it the rest of my life."

Dr. North, appearing in the doorway, white-coated as always, motioned for me to follow him. We entered an exam room. It was to be my last formal meeting with him during my therapy. He planned to leave this Friday for a vacation. I looked forward to seeing him at the support group this Wednesday, at which he was scheduled to lecture on prostate cancer.

"I still have painful, burning bowel movements," I reported. "I suspect the hc [hydrocortisone] suppositories are at least partly responsible. And I still have no diarrhea. I have a craving for salty foods such as smoked whitefish and creamed herring. I wonder if these irritate my already supersensitive bowel and anus."

"Don't worry about salty foods," he said. "They're neutralized by the time they reach the bowel. Worry only if your upper GI tract isn't okay. That is, if you have frequent indigestion and/or ulcers."

"I have some questions to ask you."

"Shoot."

"Will I need a biopsy after radiation?"

"No, unless your bone scan at that time is negative and your PSA is unusually elevated."

"What parts of my body are no longer irradiated now that we're using the conedown fields?"

"Part of the intestines. Seminal vesicles. Part of the bladder."

"Why do prostate tumors feel hard?"

"I'm not sure."

"Can it be that rapid replication crowds the space?"

"There may be some interstitial crowding. Also, the body reacts to fast or slow growth by producing collagen."

"So how am I doing?"

"Very well indeed."

"I put up a good front when I see you."

He laughed.

MAY 25. Treatment 31 of 38. It's going to be 85 degrees today, with rain possible by midday. "Better walk, you need it badly again," I tell myself. I walk, and afterwards am so achy, tired and out of sorts I want to cry. Belly swollen. Mouth hot, dry.

Anus burning. Strange aches and pains here and there. And skin threatening to crawl.

"*You* cry?" I think. "What about all the people who are much worse off than you? Quick, pop Advil and take a nap!"

Nothing unusual during today's treatment. On my back, I stared at a ceiling friend: a red patch of laser light on the lip of a small cut-out rectangle. As the linac was being set up for the frontal shot, a red laser bounced off my bifocals. I moved my head slightly to avoid it. The four large white ceiling lights made me blink. The huge machine wheezed. Mild clanking, whirring. "We're going now," said the ladies musically as they exited to be out of harm's way. What's dangerous for them, ricocheting X rays, is hopefully lifesaving for me. Squeal of the huge lead door. A red light near the ceiling far to the front of me and on my left, looking white in the corner of my vision, came on. The linac groaned, then buzzed.

After the treatment, as I donned my blue outer gown, gray-eyed Christina, twenty-five, told me about her six-year-old female quarter horse, Jessie. The tree of the western saddle, twisted to one side, had injured Jessie's back, so Christina had had to call in an expensive chiropractor vet.

MAY 26, 1993. Treatment 32 of 38. The support group met at 2:00 today in the Franklin House living room suggestive of splendorous former times. The room is so large it's more like an institutional one. Eighteen people, including five spouses and Dr. North, were present. Dr. North, tall, dignified, dark-bearded, approachable, wearing a casual gray suit and a warm smile and using good diction in a clear tenor voice, lectured with great effect. I felt proud to be his patient and to have excellent rapport with him.

"Any questions before I start?" he asked.

"Should we call it prostrate instead of prostate?" asked a woman. Her question brought laughter.

The following is essentially what he said.

If a prostate cancer cell spreads elsewhere, it's still prostate cancer. It has properties of its original site of origin. The garden variety of prostate cancer (adenocarcinoma) has a distinctive pattern of growth and spread. It tends to start as a nodule in the prostate and can infiltrate more than one lobe of the several lobes of the gland. The prostate, which sits right behind the bladder and in front of the rectum, is encapsulated by a thick fibrous tissue. The cancer can grow through the capsule and into the seminal vesicles, which are the glandular secreting organs on top of the prostate. That's all local spread, spread from the single or epicentric point into the seminal vesicles. It's one type of local-growth pattern.

Adenocarcinoma also has a propensity for spreading to the regional lymph nodes, which drain the prostate. If you have an infection or inflammation in an organ, no matter which organ it may be, appropriate lymph nodes help contain the infection or inflammation. Each organ has its own distinctive drainage pattern. The prostate, like other organs, has a well-defined pattern of lymph node drainage. The cancer invades the lymphatics within the prostate gland and has an easy passage or channel to the nodes around the prostate. Some cancer cells can invade locally. Others have a propensity to spread into the lymph nodes. And still others, by invading the prostate's capillaries, can spread systemically to other areas of the body.

The milieu the adenocarcinoma "enjoys," for lack of a better word, consists of the bones of the vertebrae, or the bones of your sacroiliac joints. Less commonly, but also involved, are the bones of the humerus and the femur. As you go out more distantly, the spread of the cancer is less common.

So, those are the most common forms of spread: the local, the regional lymph nodes, and bone. But it's not uncommon, when men have more widespread metastatic disease, for other visceral organs, like the lungs or liver, to be involved. However, that's very late in the course of the disease.

Dr. North paused. "What about staging?" someone asked.

Staging. Staging, important in making decisions regarding the treatment of the cancer, is an attempt to discover if the cancer has metastasized and, if it has, to what extent. In Stage A there's no clinical evidence of prostate cancer. The physician can't feel anything in a rectal exam. There's no nodule. The patient, however, may have symptoms of urinary obstruction and need to have a TURP, a transurethral resection of the prostate, a roto-rooter job that reams out the gland to create a wider urinary channel. When the pathologist examines the material from the gland, lo and behold he may find some prostate cancer cells. There's no clinical evidence, but there's pathological evidence from the TURP.

Stage A is further subdivided into A1 and A2. A1 indicates that there's less than 5 percent of the material from the gland that's involved with cancer. The prognosis is so favorable that we often offer no treatment, because there's only a 15 to 20 percent chance that the cancer will grow and become a clinical problem within fifteen years. Stage A2 is just like A1, but there's more than 5 percent of the tissue involved, or it's not well differentiated.

In Stage B the cancer hasn't left the gland. Stage B is prostate cancer that has grown into a nodule. You can feel it. It may have infiltrated the other lobe of the gland but it hasn't invaded the capsule, it hasn't grown through the confines of the gland. Nor has it grown to involve the seminal vesicles. It can be encompassed completely by removing the gland or irradiating it.

In Stage C the cancer has spread to nearby tissues.

In Stage D it has metastasized to nearby lymph nodes or to more distant parts of the body, often to bones.

There is controversy, unfortunately, for every stage of prostate cancer. There is no absolute best treatment for every man with Stage A or B or C or D. Patients can be treated with any or all modalities: surgery, radiation, hormonal therapy, combination therapy. The controversy for Stage A1 is whether to treat or not to treat. For A2 I would almost certainly treat. For men with Stage A2 there's an equal option of radical prostatectomy or radiation therapy, a similar cure rate of five, ten and possibly fifteen years. (By the way, surgery and

113

radiation are the only two curative modalities. Hormonal therapy is not curative; it doesn't eradicate all the cancer.)

In Stage B, between the two curative modalities, it's really a decision of the patient and the physician as to what type of morbidity (side effects) patients can deal with better. The survival rates for radical prostatectomy as against radiation are all exactly equal for Stage B, but there are different morbidities, different risks of incontinence and impotence, for example.

Stage C cannot be cured with surgery alone. If we find that a patient with B2 is upstaged to a C, pathologically, under a microscope, he needs radiation therapy afterwards. The controversy with Stage C is whether to give radiation alone, or radiation in combination with hormones.

In Stage D the tumor has spread either to the pelvic lymph nodes or to the bones. The controversy with this stage is, do we do hormonal manipulation at the initial time that we diagnose metastatic prostate cancer? Do we provide hormonal deprivation at the time of symptomatic progression? Do we try something called complete androgen deprivation, which is not only the use of an orchiectomy and/or Lupron, a drug, but the addition of other drugs, such as Eulexin? The controversy with Stage D is yes or no with hormones up front or later; and if hormones, is it complete hormones or partial ones?

A study was published in which radiation oncologists, surgeons, urologists and general internists were asked what kind of treatment they would prefer if they had Stage B cancer. The surgeons opted for a prostatectomy, the radiation oncologists for radiation—[Audience laughter.] *We preach what we practice.*

"Can you say something about Gleason numbers?" asked somebody.

Donald Gleason was a pathologist in the Veterans Administration who had a huge data bank available to him. He had thousands of prostate cancer biopsies to look at. The area where most of the cancer cells were, he gave a number of 1 to 5 and called it a major pattern. Then he looked at the minor pattern and gave that a number of 1 to 5. And he added the two together, and that's what we call a Gleason score. The 1 means it looks a lot like prostate normal tissue. The 5 means it doesn't look much like prostate tissue. The higher the combined number, the more aggressively the cells are predicted to behave. The Gleason score can range from 2 to 10. The best you can have is a 1 plus 1, the worst is a 5 plus 5.

Men with 2, 3 and 4 behave similarly, as do men with 5, 6 and 7, and men with 8, 9 and 10. The higher the Gleason score, the higher the likelihood the patient will die from prostate cancer. There are many prognostic factors in prostate cancer: age, stage, PSA, et cetera; but if you had to pick one that was the most significant prognosticator, it would be the Gleason score.

Prostate cancer, if untreated, can progress with regard to the Gleason score, and the score correlates to some degree with PSA. However, in a very high Gleason score (the 8, 9 and 10 region) the cells are often so undifferentiated, so unlike prostate normal tissue, that they no longer produce PSA, and so one can be fooled by a high Gleason score and a relatively low PSA.

Radiation oncologists are becoming more aggressive with more advanced disease. There are many different end points when we talk about prostate cancer. We can talk about overall survival. If you have a hundred men with prostate cancer today, five years later how many will be alive? Some may die of heart disease, some of stroke, some of prostate cancer, some may be hit by a truck. Some may be alive with cancer and some may be cured. So overall survival is not a good indicator of cure. You have to define what type of end point you refer to. When I talk about cure rate, I like to talk about a ten-year NED. NED stands for No Evidence of Disease. One can define a state of No Evidence of Disease; meaning, for example, someone who has just finished radiation treatment and whose prostate exam returns to normal; the nodule disappears; the PSA normalizes; there's no evidence of disease.

"What does radiation do, and why does it work?" I asked.

As you know, there are many kinds of electromagnetic radiation— radio waves, microwaves, visible light, ultraviolet light, and so on. Ionizing radiation is a type of electromagnetic radiation that has a high enough energy to expel an electron from an atom. Visible light can't expel an electron; nor can microwaves. When a high-energy X ray approaches an atom, the photon of the X ray bumps out one of the atom's outermost electrons, and that electron forms a free radical, with water, which is in the cell, and that water molecule, that hydroxyl, that free radical, attacks the DNA and causes alterations in the base pairs, or causes cuts in the strand. The cancer cell can live a long time with the DNA as is, but when the cell tries to divide and the DNA uncoils so it can self-replicate, the mitosis fails and the cell dies.

Cells that have been irradiated have been damaged. The damage is permanent, but the cell doesn't die until it tries to divide. Consequently, rapidly growing tumors, tumors that are doubling every couple of days, disappear rapidly. We irradiate them, and in a couple of days the cells go through a cell cycle and try to mitose, and they falter and die. Slow-growing tumors, like prostate cancer, which can take months to double, sometimes don't regress for a long time. If we were to biopsy a prostate after we treated it with radiation, we might find cells that look like cancer cells. They've been irradiated, they've had lethal mutations within the DNA, but they're still alive and still producing PSA. However, when they try to divide, they die. In normal prostate tissue, doubling is measured in decades. The prostate is basically nondividing tissue.

Now, why is radiation given over a period of weeks? When we provide small increments of radiation, we create sublethal amounts of DNA damage, just enough daily damage in the DNA to create one or two DNA cuts. Normal tissue, for reasons we don't understand, has the ability to repair sublethal amounts of radiation each day. Cancer cells, again for reasons unknown, do not repair sublethal amounts of radiation. So each day we add more damage to the DNA of the cancer cells, and each day, within about a four- to six-hour period, the normal tissues have repaired the DNA cut. They don't always do so, but most of the damage to the DNA is repaired quickly. As we increase the radiation dose we increase the likelihood of controlling the tumor. The larger the tumor, the larger the dose we need. And as we increase the dose, we increase the risk of major complications.

"Surgeons don't want to do surgical procedures once you've had radiation treatment. Why is that?" someone asked.

Surgeons rely a lot on normal tissues to help them with their dissection. To remove a prostate gland means dissecting part of the bladder and cutting close to the rectum. After you've been irradiated with a very high dose in that area, the tissues between the bladder, the prostate and the rectum become obscured by fibrosis, and you're at a much higher complication rate for injuries to the bladder or the rectum by the surgeon's knife. There are some surgeons who are comfortable operating in a heavily irradiated bed, and there are others who are not. If you're trained to do it, that's fine.

"Does it take longer to heal?" asked a spouse.

It can. The radiation affects small capillaries. It devitalizes them. It makes scar tissue, which is not a very vascular substance. When tissues have to heal, you want more blood to go to the capillaries and to get to the tissues faster. So, healing after surgery following radiation is delayed, prolonged, and fraught with risk.

Why radiation doesn't cause cancer is a question that's asked me quite often. You've heard for years that you have to be careful about radiation because it has carcinogenic effects. So why are you going to a radiation oncologist, who's going to blast you with radiation? The bottom line with cancer is, we do know from data from Hiroshima and Nagasaki that radiation in low doses may be carcinogenic in people who are at a stage in their life where tissues may be developing. Women who were in their adolescence in Japan in the fifteen- to twenty-year age range or thereabouts had a higher incidence of breast cancer when they were exposed to a whole-body dose of 100 rads. Low doses of radiation to women whose breasts are developing or to people whose bone marrow is actively producing cause them to be at risk for future malignancy.

The radiation we give is provided at extremely high doses. If cells are affected by the radiation, the DNA damage is lethal. We don't worry much about small mutations in the DNA, because if a target is being hit by the radiation, it's being hit by an extremely high cancer-killing dose rather than by a cancer-promoting dose. The areas we worry about are the small bits of tissue right on the edge of the radiation field. That's the area where we go rapidly from 100 percent of our dose to 0 percent. Somewhere in that range we go through a small amount of tissue that

117

does get a low dose. Consequently there are potentially cancer-causing amounts of radiation there.

Physicists and engineers have worked hard to make the distance of the falloff extremely small. Years ago, when we had a cobalt machine, we had a huge penumbra, or shadowing. It was basically an area ranging from high to medium to zero dose. Today our technologists are able to focus the X-ray beam to such an extent that the penumbra is in the order of two millimeters. We think the risk is extremely small. Cancer does occur, but it's extremely rare. It is an issue but a remote one, and the benefits of radiation far outweigh the potential risks. However, it's one of the reasons why we almost never offer radiation therapy for benign, nonmalignant diseases.

"Can you say something about PSA?" asked Harry Stengel, the group leader.

About six or seven years ago a lab in California came up with an assay that is able to measure a lipoprotein very specific to prostate cells. They called it prostate-specific antigen. Antigen means protein. It's a protein that both the normal and the malignant prostate cells produce.

The response of PSA to radiation therapy is different from the response to surgery. The level of PSA may remain elevated for a matter of weeks or months after radiation treatment. Generally, within two months we see some diminution of the PSA. This doesn't mean the cancer isn't cured. It probably means there are still malignant cells in the prostate that haven't yet gone through cell division. Generally, by six months the PSA should be normalized. Malignant cells make approximately two or three times the amount of PSA per gram of tissue that benign cells make.

If the PSA doesn't normalize by about a year after radiation we start to worry. What does normalize mean? One can have a PSA of 8 and have no cancer. [Normal is 1 to 4.] So if the PSA drops from 40 to 8 and hovers at 8 and never moves over the course of a year or a year and a half, I would call it normal for that man. At that point I would calculate a PSA density just to make sure the volume of his prostate would indicate having that high a PSA.

PSA density is the value of PSA divided by the volume of the prostate. It's a number that gives you a relative suspicion of the likelihood of cancer. The lower the PSA density, the more likely you are to have a normal prostate.

PSA closely correlates with the volume and stage of cancer. As the volume of the malignant cells rises and takes up a larger portion of the gland, the higher the stage and the higher the PSA. The amount of cancer cells within the body closely correlates with the PSA. If you have benign prostatic hypertrophy (BPH), it means you have an enlarged gland. Such a gland will produce a higher PSA. A PSA of 20 makes me worried there's cancer.

When a man dies at the age of sixty for reasons other than prostate cancer, at autopsy there's about a 50 percent chance you'll find prostate cancer. The risk increases about 1 percent each year.

"I'm sorry I have to leave," I said, rising. "I have a radiation date." General laughter. "It's a great lecture. Thanks very much," I added, shaking Dr. North's hand.

MAY 27. Treatment 33 of 38. With today I will have had almost 87 percent of my therapy. This morning, glancing into a large mirror at my naked body, I was startled to see I had almost no pubic hair, and I could now easily make out the three tatoo marks. I had felt the increasing absence of pubic hair while showering lately, but the sight of its absence came as a fresh surprise. My groin amusingly resembled that of a preadolescent.

I asked the two Maries this afternoon if my pubic hair will grow back. They assured me it will, although Marie Whiteson said, "It may come back blond."

"Are you kidding?"

"Sometimes people get different hair from what they had," said Marie Izant. "Straight if it was curly. Curly if it was straight. Black if it was blond."

"I'm thinking of starting a business in pubic-hair wigs," I said.

119

As I was on my way to the dressing room after my treatment, nurse Tanya O'Neill, standing behind the high nurses' counter, asked, "How're you doing? Any diarrhea?"

"No. But my nights are disturbed by frequent painful peeing, and I find myself getting angry at parts of my body."

"That's understandable. Do you have a metallic taste in your mouth?"

"Come to think of it, I do."

"Many people report that. Especially those who have radiation in the head area."

"I think my taste buds may be affected, and that that's why I have a craving for strong-tasting foods."

MAY 28, 1993, FRIDAY MORNING. Treatment 34 of 38. The past three days, especially the mornings, have been rough. My sleep is disturbed by frequent, painful urination. Bowel movements are also painful; afterwards I feel as if I have the flu. And I have the damnedest aches and pains. The side effects seem relentless. Will they ever let up? Clearly, they worsen the longer the therapy continues. Well, I don't have long to go: four treatments after today, and I will have had almost 90 percent of my therapy behind me!

Last night I awoke with the usual metallic taste in my mouth, and my gums felt strange, as if I hadn't flossed in months. As I descended the stairs on my way to the kitchen for something to cool my hot mouth, my right thigh ached badly. "What's causing *this* ache? And why is my right shoulder blade hurting badly?" I wondered. I tried a spoonful of vanilla ice cream. Wrong medicine. A sip of bitter lemon. Wrong again. I retreated to my bed, where I sat in the dark a while, stretching arms, feet and legs in an effort to get my body to feel normal. I gave up and tried to sleep, and finally succeeded.

It's not easy to concentrate on work when you feel you have the flu. You move about creakily. What to do? Read the paper?

The *Times* ought to have a day when it emphasizes good news in an effort to counteract all the usual bad. I'm a phony at the Oncology Center, all smiles, jokes and gaiety.

This afternoon, as I turned to open the door of the men's dressing room, I saw again the man with the bloated-looking skin. He was wearing a white hospital gown, and walking very slowly on crutches toward the waiting room. Bald, tan head; hunched, frail shoulders; thin, brown, shiny, hairless legs in brown socks and in the scuffed brown moccasin shoes of yesterday.

"When's your last day?" I asked him later, in the waiting room. A pause. He seemed uncertain about whether he wanted to engage in conversation. A shy, reserved man, but maybe only because of pain.

"Tuesday."

"When did you have the full treatment?"

He frowned uncertainly. "Four or five years ago."

"Did you have burning urination?"

"No. I wore a tube for four months. With a bag. I had an obstruction."

"In your urethra?"

"I think in my prostate."

"Caused by the radiation?"

"I'm not sure. Then I had a T-U-R. I was reamed out," he added in case I didn't understand his meaning. He meant a TURP. "After that I urinated through my penis."

"No problem with surgery after radiation?"

"No. I have thirty-eight tumors. Vertebrae. Legs. Across my chest. Right side of my head."

"What's bone pain like? Is it like bad muscular pain?" He smiled ruefully. "Like joint pain?"

"It's bad. . . ."

"Does radiation help?"

"It shrinks the tumors. . . . Kills them. . . . The pain goes away."

121

His name being called, he gathered his crutches and a white canvas bag, causing a swaying in the large black rectangular box, dangling on his chest, that was supported by a black strap around his neck. On rising, he let out a sudden, brief, sharp cry of pain. "My back hurts," he said in embarrassment without glancing at me, and made his slow, awkward way out of the small room into which Vivaldi's *The Four Seasons* was being piped. Soft, gentle voice. Round cheeks. Shiny legs. Large, sad eyes. "The troubles they've seen," I thought. "Poor, brave man. What keeps him going? A wife? Children? Grandchildren? Is there a car waiting for him?" I felt like crying.

"Do you have patients with testicular cancer?" I asked the two Maries as I lay on my back on the twenty-thousand-dollar patient's table.

"Not at present," replied Marie Whiteson. "It's mostly guys in their twenties."

"High cure rate," said Marie Izant.

"Really?" I asked, surprised. "I read somewhere it's a tough one."

"They usually have one testicle removed," said Marie Izant.

"So what are you going to do this long weekend?" asked Marie Whiteson as I left the table and started to put on my blue gown.

"I'm going to rest. What about you?"

"I'll be glad to just be quiet."

"And you?" I asked Marie Izant.

"Oh, she," said Marie Whiteson. "She'll be in Wildwood."

"Wildwood," I groaned. "That crazy place."

Smiling, Marie Izant spread her arms wide. "I'm going to get some sun!" she cried.

MAY 30, 1993, SUNDAY. This has been a rough week for me. I feel increasingly tired, maybe because I walked four of the days. Joan advises me to walk more slowly and less far. Burning urination. Burning anus. She took charge of me today, emphasizing low-bulk diet, mild foods, lots of rest. One more week to go! And a short one at that, tomorrow being a holiday. Get thee behind me, prostate cancer! I'm looking forward to a new life, a life after radiation therapy. But what if I'm *not* cured? What then? And what if I have permanent side effects?

JUNE 2, 1993, WEDNESDAY. Treatment 36 of 38. Yesterday nurse Debby Kuban said, "You don't need another complete blood count, because you'll be finished with therapy on Friday. See? That's proof you're coming to the end." I'll have had a total of 6840 rads (180 daily times 38). Will I recover from burning urination and burning rectum and anus? What about the possibility of ulceration of bladder and bowel? And what will my PSA be a month after therapy?

Mornings are the worst time, because of bowel movements. Even on a low-bulk diet, I have two or three each morning, and the anus burns fiercely both during the movement and for a couple of hours afterwards. The pain is fatiguing. Resting in the lounger afterwards, I feel my anus pulsing with pain. A couple of Advils, taken with cranberry juice diluted with water, help in about an hour.

The oncoming of a bowel movement is itself unpleasant, and very different from a normal oncoming one. I feel a pervasive, increasing malaise, then increasing anxiety. Only later do I feel signals in the bowel, which come suddenly and urgently while my sphincter warns me I lack normal control over it. Nor do I have the usual control over how much I can eliminate. Something abruptly shuts down the procedure though I know there's more to come, and experiments have taught me that squeezing will only do harm.

(I'm discussing these very intimate matters, and at some length, in the hope my doing so may be helpful to other patients.)

One of my side effects is gastrointestinal disturbance—a difficulty in digesting, and a lack of harmony between my appetite and my ability to digest. I've lost my perspective about food. This became obvious when I went wild over salty things: smoked whitefish, creamed herring, smoked tuna; as well as over canned whipped cream and, later, heavy whipping cream. My current intake of high-cholesterol foods is clearly inadvisable, but it's temporary and helps lessen the feeling of acidity throughout my digestive system. However, it fails to eliminate the metallic taste in my mouth.

I'm reminded of Bernie Breitbart's mother, who was in her early eighties when her doctor warned her to lower her cholesterol count. "Is he *crazy?*" she said passionately to Bernie after the medical visit. She died of other causes not too long afterwards.

In the Oncology Center waiting room this afternoon I was more jumpy than usual, and a little sick to my stomach. It occurred to me I may have become therapy gun-shy. In the beginning I welcomed the linear accelerator as my potential savior, but now that I may be "cured," whatever the word means in the present context, it's possible I fear the inner roasting. Also, I may be experiencing withdrawal symptoms, which if true would not be surprising inasmuch as I've received lots of attention for almost eight weeks from a number of very pleasant, even affectionate people.

JUNE 4, 1993, FRIDAY. Treatment 38 of 38. My last treatment day! As I prepared to leave the house for the Oncology Center, "I need to pee," warned my bladder.

"No!" I responded firmly. "You peed on schedule just fifteen minutes ago! You know you're not allowed to pee again! Why are you so perverse? Quit bugging me!"

In the dressing room the locker doors were all ajar. So was the restroom door. And the restroom light was on. How enticing the restroom looked! I was tempted to pee. After all, this was my last day. So what if my bladder got zapped a bit?

"No!" said an inner voice. "There's also discipline to consider!" So I held it in. By the time I was on the table, waiting for the first zap, my need to pee had become urgent. *Only four zaps. Don't linger afterwards. No Russian good-byes. Head straight for the restroom john.*

"You're married, aren't you?" asked Marie Izant.

"Yes."

"Do you ever bring your wife?"

"No."

"Why not?"

"What would I want her here for?"

She laughed.

"My pubic hair is coming back," I remarked.

"Oh yeah?" said Joy Engelson idly.

"It's coming back blue," I said.

"No, red," said dark-haired Marie Whiteson jokingly.

"Is there much burnout here? Are you ladies depressed by what you see?"

"Not really," said Marie Izant.

"We have a high cure rate," Marie Whiteson said.

Suddenly, with a swift, expert gesture Marie Whiteson removed my adhesived name tag from the conedown block before slipping the block out of the machine, whose muzzle at the moment was above me.

"You're getting rid of me," I said.

"Aren't you glad to be finished?"

"Yes, but I'll miss you ladies. You've been wonderful. The morale here is very high. I'm sure it helps the healing process."

Leaving the table, with Marie Izant's help I placed my body cast into a large plastic sack I had brought for the occasion. I wanted to study it away from the superprofessional treatment room. Now for the bathroom! But as I left the treatment room, I was called aside by Christina to look at some photos of her horse Jessie she had brought especially to show me. When I finished looking at them I realized the other techs were busy with another patient and that I hadn't said good-bye. Which was just as well, I told myself, for my eyes felt teary. I had become attached to the young ladies, and it wasn't easy to divorce myself from them.

The bathroom was empty. What a relief to lift my two gowns and pee! Nothing to do now but relax, change, leave the building, and begin a new journey to recover from the side effects of the old.

Two weeks ago, having forgotten how dreary I feel every Friday after five successive days of radiation, I invited Bernie Breitbart and Alison Harris, housemates, to join Joan and me for dinner this evening to celebrate my graduation. But today I wasn't up to eating anything, or even to just going out. Some of my soft tissues, the ones that feel they've been barbecued, are emulating my creaking bones. So I called Bernie in the afternoon and apologetically postponed the dinner.

Joan congratulated me on finishing therapy. So did Susy. So did friend Kate, calling from Santa Cruz. So did Cousin Erik. I'm grateful for these calls. I've been feeling cut off lately, for some reason. My invalidism?

Eight

June 11 to July 17, 1993

JUNE 11, 1993, FRIDAY. Today is a week since my final treatment. I've done my part by undergoing radiation therapy. Now, soon, a month after therapy, I'll see what radiation therapy has done for me, because that's when I'll have my first post-therapy PSA. Dr. North once told me, "I used to take my patients' PSA during therapy. And I'd have a heart attack, because, as it turned out, it rises during radiation. So I stopped taking it. Since then I do it a month after therapy, and every three months thereafter for about a year."

What will my number be? I recall that it was 16.4 before I began therapy. So now will it be 12? 11? After all, I have a very large gland, which generates a lot of PSA. Be thankful for small favors, I caution myself. Don't ask for too much. Don't, through greed or hubris, bring down upon yourself Jehovah's wrath.

I try not to think about the number but I can't help doing it. PSA is like a clerk in a great court sitting in judgment on me, on my health or illness, my life or death. What terrible or wonderful message will this clerk deliver? Will I be condemned? Or rescued? And will the tumor be smaller? If so, how small? Will my side effects have been experienced in vain? Did I make a serious mistake in not selecting a prostatectomy? Or watchful waiting? Wait, wait, wait and see.

I sense some side effect improvement, especially in peeing, which is less painful, yet at night I have the same old difficulty:

127

getting up frequently, and with trouble starting and ending the stream. It's hard to predict how I may feel at any one moment. I think I'm more peppy; then suddenly I poop out, and I feel so exhausted I imagine I'm close to death; and then, miraculously, I recover enough to work on my journal or move about. I haven't done my power walk for eleven days; my body warns against it.

I'm getting fed up with all the mild foods, especially the heavy creams, I've been ingesting to spare rectum and anus. I'm going off the creams today, which make me feel infantile. I dislike even the suggestion of feeling or acting like an invalid.

Cousin Erik called this evening. He saw his urologist, Fledermaus, yesterday and finally (at my urging) learned his Gleason score: 6, the same as mine. True, it's not 2, 3 or 4, but I still believe Fledermaus sold him a bill of goods when he assured him that at his age (Erik was seventy-one at the time) only a radical prostatectomy is a cure for prostate cancer.

JUNE 12. This morning something happened that hadn't occurred in weeks: I didn't have a bowel movement. I take this as a sign of some bowel recovery. The mental uplift I receive from not having a movement is accompanied by a substantial physical one. Not only am I spared the pain as of being burned by an acid; I'm also rewarded by a return of some of my old energy. I'm beginning to regain body heat, which was conspicuously absent during therapy. Peeing is no longer urgent, difficult and frequent. The stream is better, and the burning has greatly subsided. Also, I no longer have the metallic taste in my mouth. What's particularly interesting about these three events (my not having a bowel movement, my not having frequent and painful urination, and my not being tired and cold much of the time) is that they occurred in a quantum leap: I received no warning of their coming.

Joan, familiar with my curiosity about scientific and technological subjects, brought to my attention a couple of days ago that today there would be an open house at the Princeton Plasma Physics Laboratory (PPPL), a facility of the U.S. Department of Energy, where for more than forty years scientists and engineers have tried to produce significant amounts of energy through controlled fusion, the method by which the sun and other stars produce their energy. My friend and neighbor, Bernie Breitbart, and I went, and toured the place.

Spacious grounds: lawns, trees, plantings. A low, long brick building suggesting an affluent public school. Huge, boxlike buildings. Rows of what looked like Quonset huts. Things resembling groups of trailer trucks. Inside some of the buildings the scale was laughably large. A control room, with banks of computers, made me think of a flight to Mars. In another building were weird, curving, curling, disappearing, mind-blowing pipes.

We joined a crowd watching demonstrations of the effects of extremely low temperatures, which struck me as quaint inasmuch as one of the chief aims of PPPL is to reach and sustain for a whole second a temperature of a hundred million degrees Celsius. (The temperature of the interior of the sun is estimated to be fifteen million degrees Celsius). A man with a foreign accent, wearing a tag reading "Dr. Zero," bounced a pink rubber ball on a table, then on the floor. He inserted the ball into a container of liquid nitrogen. On removing it he dropped it from a height. It hit the table top with the thud of a billiard ball. He tossed three green grapes into a styrofoam cup of liquid nitrogen. The grapes, being relatively hot, caused the liquid to boil and "steam." He suspended the heads of some daisies into a styrofoam cup of liquid nitrogen, removed them with a thick, elbow-length glove and, making a fist, crushed them into a white powder.

A young man, Dr. Zero's assistant, lighting a kitchen match, placed its yellow flame above a tank of vaporizing liquid nitrogen. The flame promptly died, the vapor (gaseous nitrogen) having shoved aside the oxygen necessary to sustain combustion. The young man displayed the lack of springiness, at room temperature, of a long lead spring suspending a weight; and of its springiness immediately after it had been cooled in a bath of liquid nitrogen. There were other demonstrations, among them a tiny example of magnetic levitation.

During our visit I had no problem with fatigue. And I ate a frankfurter and some salty chips and twirls, with no aftereffects of burping or heartburn.

JUNE 14. I'm restless, eager to move about, take a walk, but I had a relapse today. Three bowel movements; rectal discomfort; anal pain; great fatigue. The weather was lovely, but I was too tired and brittle to do anything but work a little and read. I was depressed and disgruntled most of the day, much more so than when I was having therapy. I want badly to quit being a prisoner of bowel movements. And I'm tired of walking on eggshells.

This prostate cancer business has screwed up my relations with the seasons. Because I have less body heat than normal, I'm obliged to wear clothes heavier than is appropriate for the time of year. I want to return as promptly as possible to appropriateness. It's fatiguing to constantly feel out of step and tune. Also, a problem in illness is that I tend to concentrate too much on my body's language. If I listen intently enough to my bodily functions they'll increase their decibel levels to please me.

What if I never return to "normal"? In that case I'll have to become better acquainted with the new person I've become. High time I started self-hypnosis in an effort to improve my recovery from side effects and to try to kill any lingering cancer cells. The high-energy X rays kill some of the cancer cells outright and kill many by interfering with mitosis, but it's by no means certain some cells don't survive to produce new colonies. Time to help the body with the use of mind. I'm reminded that back in 1980, the year in which, coincidentally, I first began to worry about having prostate cancer, I had a successful experience with self-hypnosis.

JUNE 19, 1993. It's now two weeks since the completion of my therapy. Despite some ups and downs, I'm feeling much better. I've resumed my power walks and am working well. I took my walk very early this morning to avoid the heat. We have a record heat for this day: 95 degrees in New York, 102 degrees in Newark.

I met today with Edward Helmschrott, the medical physicist of the King City radiation oncology team, in his office at the Oncology Center. As the reader knows, I was very curious, for some reason, about almost every aspect of prostate cancer— the disease itself, and the various treatments of it—so it was not surprising that my curiosity led me to interview him about his work. What did a medical physicist *do*? And what was his relationship to the rest of the radiation oncology staff? He was an energetic man in his early forties, with a large black mustche and an altogether pleasant manner. The following is essentially what he said.

Let me begin by going back to the opening of our clinic here. The first step was to select the equipment. I analyzed the technical aspects of the equipment and Dr. Mapleton, our chief physician here, checked its practical aspects. We needed a linear accelerator to provide the treatments; also a radiation therapy simulator, which has the same geometry as a linear accelerator but produces pictures that are much more visually acute. The linear accelerator makes such high-energy X rays that the images it produces are poor; whereas the radiation therapy simulator uses a standard (lower energy) X-ray tube, which, though it's unsuitable for treating cancer, produces superb images.

Once we decided on the type of equipment, we selected a linear accelerator that produces two different X-ray energy beams: a 6 MV [million electron volts] and a 15 MV, plus five different electron-beam energies. Electrons are totally different from X rays. X rays are pure electromagnetic energy. Electrons are actually charged particles, with mass. They penetrate much less deeply in normal soft tissue than X rays do, so they're very good in treating superficial tumors, where you can deliver a high dose near the surface and a lower dose to healthy tissues underneath. With such different characteristics in mind, we had many different options to consider.

After we selected our equipment, I had to design the shielding. The linear accelerator is encased in a concrete bunker, with walls as thick as five feet in certain places. The ceiling is also shielded. The reason is, some of the high-energy X rays will be absorbed by the patient; others will pass through the patient, scatter around the room and will eventually exit unless you provide enough shielding to contain them. Every time they bounce, they lose energy. But some of the X rays have so much energy, they can ricochet a few times and still have enough energy to penetrate a foot or two of concrete.

"Are you saying that if the lead door of the treatment room isn't shut, the X rays can leave the room and go elsewhere?" I asked.

Correct. The reason we have that narrow passage, that maze, is so the radiation has to bounce around before it can make it through the maze to strike the door. Also, since it has ricocheted a few times and lost some energy, we don't need as heavy a door as we otherwise would. As it is, that door has three-quarter-inch lead throughout its entire surface, with maybe another three to four inches of heavy plastic.

"What's its weight? A thousand pounds?"

I would imagine a lot more.

"By the time the radiation reaches the prostate, beginning with 15 million electron volts, how much energy do we have?"

That number refers to the speed of the electrons before they strike the target. When X rays were first discovered at the turn of the century, they were produced by accelerating electrons between a potential difference; that is, between a negative electrode and a positive one. If you put 70 thousand volts across those two electrodes, the electrons would travel at a certain velocity when striking the target, and the strength, so to speak, of the X rays would be different than if you had 100 thousand volts between the two electrodes. You can probably build a machine that has maybe as much as a million electron volts between two electrodes before you get to shielding and insulation problems. If you actually had 15 million volts between two electrodes, you couldn't go anywhere near the machine, because you wouldn't have enough insulation to prevent the voltage from leaving its desired path and maybe hitting someone.

The linear accelerator produces X rays somewhat differently; that is, in the way the electrons are accelerated. Microwaves are used to speed up the electrons. Now, we have a tungsten target, which is basically a chunk of tungsten containing some water channels to cool it. When the electrons strike the target, X rays are produced. As the X rays pass through the patient's body some are absorbed, some are deflected and some just pass through. As they penetrate each centimeter of tissue, more and more X rays are attenuated. The radiation damage inflicted on the cells is produced by secondary electrons released by the X rays. As an X ray hits the surface of the skin, it releases electrons, which travel a certain distance before they impart damage. The higher the X-ray energy striking the skin, the deeper the initial burst of damage. It's called the depth of maximum dose.

"Does the machine leak radiation laterally?"

There is some leakage from the general vicinity of the target, but it's small and is limited by state regulations.

"So if you didn't have a concrete bunker, leaking radiation would injure people?"

If the same person sat at a desk the other side of, let's say a plasterboard wall, day in, day out, that would be true. But if you had a facility out in the middle of nowhere, with the closest occupied space being five or six hundred yards away, you could reduce your shielding, because by the time the radiation reached that person its intensity would be low.

"The technicians enter the treatment room soon after the machine stops buzzing, so apparently the energy dissipates fairly rapidly."

Yes.

"Are you also involved in the machine's maintenance?"

I measure the radiation beams and the different characteristics after the machine is initially built. We refer to this as the initial commissioning of the machine. It's a process that can take from a month to two months, depending on the number of X-ray beams the machine will

133

produce. Once we characterize the beams, I have an ongoing quality-insurance testing program, in which I monitor certain characteristics at various time intervals to make sure they haven't changed.

"Are you happy with the machine?"

Yes.

"Do you ever work with cancer patients directly?"

Only when we introduce radioactive materials inside of a patient to treat certain types of tumors. In that case I and one of the physicians implant the devices.

"They're in the form of needles or pellets?"

Yes.

"What's your typical day here like?"

I'm involved with various hospital committees regarding radiation safety, and there are administrative and bureaucratic things I need to do. I keep up with various state and federal regulations and with various ongoing seminars. I lecture to technical groups within the hospital. I organize the machine's maintenance. I answer any specific questions a physician or a technologist may have regarding a patient's treatment. And so on. Such things keep me busy.

Patients are referred to us either by a chemotherapist or a medical oncologist. The patient has already been diagnosed with the disease, so we know what we're dealing with. The physician examines the patient and recommends a course of treatment. We set up a simulation, in which the patient is placed in the treatment position; and, using the radiotherapy simulator, the physician zeros in on the anatomy he wishes to treat, and decides what basic technique he's going to use. At that point we get either CT images or manual contours of the part of the patient's body to be treated. We put that information into our treatment planning computer, and at that point I get involved.

I input the data into our planning computer, which simulates what the doses inside the patient will be, based on his or her characteristics. There are various factors: the size of the patient, the patient's contours, the size of the radiation beam, the angles at which the beams will enter the body, and any beam-modifying devices to be used in the particular treatment. All these can affect the dose distribution within the body.

"Also the prostate's size?"

No. The internal makeup of the body has very little effect, because at such a high energy the interaction between the energy and different types of tissues is almost identical. The shape of the body would have a larger effect.

"Body mass or body fat?"

Just the shape. For example, some abdomens are square, others are curvy. Some have a greater distance between their prostate and their anterior surface. All these characteristics can affect the distribution of the intensity inside the body. Our computer simulates them and shows us where the highest and lowest intensities are, and what the distribution is with regard to the location of the gland and the surrounding lymph nodes. After I come up with a number of plans of attack, I discuss them with the physician and he selects one. At that point we write the directions into the chart for the technologists to follow. Then we do calculations to determine how long the machine has to stay on to deliver the desired dose. In order to come up with the precise amount of time, we use the various characteristics I've measured.

"In terms of lethal radiation, for example the kind that occurred at Chernobyl, what comparable levels are we dealing with? I've heard the human body can accept much more energy locally than across the whole body. Is that correct?"

Yes. We usually don't refer to energy when we're discussing things of that nature. We refer to the dose, because you can deliver equivalent doses with both high- and low-energy X rays. At Chernobyl the radiation-producing isotopes were fission-reaction products. Their energies were much, much lower than that produced by the linear accelerator. But the intensity and the amount of radioactive material were so high that the doses delivered were very, very high. The radiation produced in our linear accelerator is made electronically. The X rays produced in the accelerator originate from electrons released from a hot-wire filament. These electrons are accelerated by a microwave energy on their way to the target. Turn off the power, and the X-ray production stops.

At Chernobyl you had physical radioactive material. The radiation emitted from the material could strike you and give you a certain dose.

Or your body could ingest the material and you could have the radiation source inside your body. Such radiation doesn't stop until the radioactive material decays to a very low level. So there are two totally different sources of radiation: the linear accelerator and a radioactive material. The Chernobyl kind is more deadly because you can ingest it and can't get rid of it.

"I understand you use Cerrobend for making blocks because it has a low melting point."

Right. It's an alloy of lead, tin, bismuth and cadmium, and has a very low melting point but a very high density: 90 percent of the density of lead. It produces a nice, compact piece of metal that absorbs a lot of radiation and allows us to cast blocks in a variety of shapes, with relatively little danger to the person making the casting. Cerrobend is the trade name of a particular metal produced by one company. There are several companies, and depending on the mixture of the four different components, the melting point might be slightly higher or lower.

"The reason for using Cerrobend is because it's possible to process it in-house?"

Yes. You could cast lead blocks, but you'd need a very hot oven to melt the lead, and a form that could withstand the temperature, and you'd have to somehow machine the form to the shape the physician prescribes. Because this alloy has a very low melting point, we can cast it inside styrofoam blocks. All we need is a hot-wire device to cut the shape in the styrofoam, and then we can make a casting in a matter of minutes.

"What's the physics of the damage to cancer cells?"

With X rays the damage to the cell is delivered by secondary electrons. An atom is composed of a nucleus and orbiting electrons, and these are physical, charged particles. When the radiation interacts with an atom, electrons are ejected, and they produce an ionization track that's very dense, much denser than an X ray. What these ionizations do is disrupt the chemistry in the cancer cells' DNA. We may not kill the cell outright but we can damage it, so the next time it tries to divide it fails and then dies. In order to kill tumor cells directly with an X-ray beam, you'd need a very high dose, much higher than normal tissues can tolerate. Since cancer cells divide much more rapidly than benign ones, if you damage them to the point where if they try to divide they die, you've accomplished the same thing, yet you're sparing the normal tissues, since the latter divide much less frequently.

JUNE 23, 1993. While shaving this morning I thought, "What if the radiation gets rid of cancer cells in the way my razor removes my beard; that is, without getting at the underlying cause? Maybe in five years a new cancer-beard will emerge. If I die of other causes before then, my radiation therapy will be regarded as a cure. If you give radiation therapy to an eighty-five-year-old man, he's almost certainly going to be 'cured.'"

There was a support group meeting in the afternoon, this time in a much smaller room of the Franklin House in King City. Nine people were present, including a woman, Barbara, John Darrough's wife. Morton Blumberg, 75, stout, gray-bearded, outgoing, was full of information regarding doctors, treatments and nostrums. Diagnosed with prostate cancer in August 1986, he had radiation therapy. The cancer has recurred, and hormone therapy has made him impotent. He believes shark cartilage, taken orally, is good for prostate cancer, and he bought $2000 worth of the stuff in Florida.

"It costs $145 for five grams. They last about six days," he said. "A woman friend told me her house water made her husband's PSA go up a number of points."

"Water doesn't affect PSA," I said.

A pause as Blumberg studied me. "Oh, I forgot," he said. "He had a urinary infection. The water in the house was full of orgasms." Another pause. "Orgasms? . . . What am I saying?" he added, and laughed nervously. "Orgasms. . . . That's in the past. . . . I meant organisms." Despite his gray beard I could see he was reddening.

George Henry reported he's having a hard time with his cancer. "Three TURPs in six months!" he said loudly, frowning. "My tumor is four inches long and is pressing against my bladder.

There's some bleeding, and possibly blood clots. But my current PSA is normal: 3.2. I obviously can't continue with this. My next regimen will probably be chemotherapy." Like two or three other members of the group, he reported having had bad experiences at Memorial Sloan-Kettering Cancer Center in New York. "Big Apple," he remarked acidly.

"Like cattle in a cattle chute," said Pete Wayne, a minister, to me drily in an aside.

Buzzing of little pill containers. Morton Blumberg laughed empathetically. Harry Stengel, the group leader, who had a small plastic bottle of water on a table beside him, swallowed a little water while downing a pill.

"I've noticed that since my orchiectomy my wife does things a lot faster," said Henry Lombardi. "I wonder if it has anything to do with my impotence."

"Now that you mention it, I think *my* wife does the same thing," said Stengel. "You wonder how spouses feel about it. By the way, I'm still looking into possibly having an orchiectomy."

"*My* wife doesn't care. Make money! That's it!" said Blumberg. "Just kidding," he added softly, smiling.

A number of men in the group were impotent, and they seemed to believe nothing could be done about their impotence, but when I said, "There are ways of causing an erection," Harry Stengel asked, "You mean by injection?" and made a painful face. He was referring to injecting the penis.

"They implant a rod in the penis," somebody said. "Not a rod," said another man. "It's supposed to be able to go down." Laughter.

"It's a silicone implant, with an interior pump," I said. "My cousin has a friend who's had great success with one. He got married soon after it was implanted."

"What about silicone? Isn't the government worried?" somebody asked.

I told about Cousin Erik's experience with the noninvasive vacuum device.

"How long does the erection last?" asked Harry Stengel.

"Twenty minutes, I think."

"Well, we develop other interests as we age," said Morton Blumberg.

"My brother was impotent in his fifties!" cried John Darrough. "Result of a prostatectomy! Ten years later he said to me, 'I *wondered* if something was wrong!'"

More laughter.

"Can you have an orgasm after a prostatectomy?" a voice asked.

"It's called a dry orgasm. There's no semen, no fluid," responded another voice.

"What about after a TURP?"

"Some men have retrograde ejaculations after a TURP. It doesn't come out. It goes into the bladder," said Henry Lombardi.

"This meeting has been more intimate than most," said Stengel softly, with a shy smile, as the meeting was about to end.

"It's because the room is much smaller," Barbara Darrough said.

JUNE 25. Today is three weeks since I finished therapy, and I'm daily feeling stronger and I no longer have painful urination and bowel movements. My first inkling that I was improving was the radical decline in the number of bowel movements. I felt uplifted, almost elated, on the day when I had only one. To an outsider this may seem like excessive anal interest. To me it was an important signal that helped allay my chief anxiety: permanent rectal injury; possibly rectal surgery; even, possibly (though unlikely, given the percentages), a colostomy.

I avoid spicy foods to spare my inflamed insides and because such foods cause painful urination and bowel movements. I also indulge in heavy (whipping) cream to soothe the inner roasted areas, and lots of Jello, either ready-made or made in quantity by Joan.

Sylvia, of my Cibachrome class, arrived at my house at 9:00 A.M. and I drove us to the Met in New York to see "The Waking Dream," an exhibition based on the first century of photography. We interrupted our viewing with lunch at the Met and a brief outdoor excursion, then finished looking at the large exhibition, composed of 253 works. We returned to Princeton at about 8:00 P.M. and I wasn't at all tired, an obvious sign I'm improving.

JULY 2, 1993, FRIDAY. Four weeks since I finished therapy. I called Harry Stengel, a fine, gentle man, this afternoon, and we chatted about his condition. His cancer was diagnosed when he was seventy-one. His Gleason grade was 4+4. "Until then I felt very good," he said. "I looked forward to having many fine years ahead of me, and to doing various things. It all suddenly changed. Lord." He goes to Colorado tomorrow for two weeks. I'm to phone him a couple of days after his return and make a date to interview him about his case.

JULY 5, 1993. I've been walking and socializing normally, and making various smalls trips by car. I spent the July 4th weekend with Erik and Molly in Irvington, New York, where they live. The village, named after Washington Irving, contains Sunnyside, a house and estate overlooking the Hudson, where he lived. We went to the Neuberger Museum at SUNY (State University of New York) in Purchase, where I was startled by the beauty of an exhibition of carved wooden bowls. In the evening Erik played for me an explicit videotape showing the operation of the vacuum device for obtaining an erection. He still feels it's not for him; too painful.

Cancer cells are disorderly, multiply rapidly and, if left unchecked, often destroy the host. In doing so they destroy themselves. Benign tumors usually don't destroy the host; they're content to live in partnership. If they destroy the host, it's not because it's their intention to do so. It may happen incidentally because of their large size. When viewed through a microscope, cancer cells lose their normal appearance and seem to indulge in antic, eccentric behavior. Do they have an identity crisis? They certainly cause the host to have one. I read at the medical library that on some occasions certain cancer cells, resistant to irradiation, form "daughter" colonies. Why daughter? Has the notion of *femme fatale* invaded studies of prostate cancer?

An epidemiological study of this cancer, published in *JAMA* (the *Journal of the American Medical Association*) of May 26, 1993, concluded, based on the fact that survival rates appear, currently, to be unchanging, that essentially there are three current treatment modalities: (1) radical prostatectomy, (2) high-energy radiation, and (3) watchful waiting. What was lacking, perhaps necessarily, given the broad-based nature of the study, is the difference between chronological and physiological age. All men are not created physiologically equal, nor do they age equally. To advise that a radical prostatectomy should not be performed on men over 75 may be useful in most cases, but it overlooks the fact that some 75-year-olds may be closer to 65 physiologically. Also, watchful waiting may affect the quality of life of certain imaginative patients, who might strain to hear the once-secret ticking of a time bomb.

JULY 6. This afternoon I had blood drawn at the hospital for a PSA and an acid phosphatase, and I'll get the results from Dr. North when I meet with him on the 12th. What will my PSA be? What's happening in my prostate? Are cancer cells trying to divide? Is the tumor disappearing? Is the gland shrinking? Will Dr. North do a digital? If he does, what will he find? Will he be surprised? Pleased? Disappointed? How will I feel?

JULY 12, 1993. I went to the Oncology Center, changed into a hospital gown and walked toward the waiting room. Dr. North, wearing the usual long white coat, was writing something as he stood before the high counter at the nurses' station. "There's the man," I said affectionately.

Turning to me with a broad smile, he said, "Your PSA's excellent. I'll be with you shortly," and strode down the corridor.

Feeling grateful to him for giving me the good news *at once* (many people, consciously or otherwise, tend to withhold information because knowledge is power), I began to relax after the long weeks of suspense, and chatted with nurses Tanya O'Neill and Debby Kuban before taking a seat in the waiting room, where everything seemed to have brightened because my news was good.

"I haven't seen you before," said an older man in a hospital gown, addressing me. There was one other person in the room, an elderly woman in a tight-fitting white turban and a yellow gown. "I have two weeks to go," he said. "I heard it gets harder toward the end. A man here last week had thirty-seven treatments. He said he didn't think he could take one day more."

The man was called away. The woman, sitting opposite me, was riffling through a magazine. Her eyebrows had been thinly painted on. Her eyes with their prominent upper lids looked tired. Sandals revealed almost black big-toe nails. Her shanks shone with blotchy brown skin.

"They told me I had six months," she said in a flat voice. "That was three years ago."

"What do you have?"

"Liver and pancreas. They tried chemotherapy. My liver hurts." She placed her right hand over where I took her appendix to be. "They switched to radiation."

I felt sad for her; and helpless. And contrasted her state with mine. The luck of the draw. Einstein has been quoted as saying, "I don't believe God plays dice with the universe," meaning he believed the universe isn't chaotic, without fundamental laws. I sometimes, as now, wondered if God plays dice with us humans. I noticed Dr. North in the doorway, waiting for me.

"Do you want to know your PSA?" he asked in the exam room.

"Yes."

"8.9."

"Is that good?"

"It's excellent. It's almost half what it was when I first saw you: 16.4. I'm very happy about it. I believe it's the largest drop I've seen in any of my patients a month after therapy." He put his head back and stared at the ceiling, squinting with thought.

"How's my acid phosphatase?"

"Slightly elevated. 3.9. We expect it to be elevated if the prostate is inflamed. Normal is up to 3.8. I don't put much stock in phosphatase now that we have PSA. PSA is very specific. I ordered a phosphatase for you because I didn't have one in my files. I expect your PSA will continue to go down for some time."

"When will I see you again?"

"In three months."

"I'm going to California in mid-August and will return around the middle of October. Is there a problem in my going?"

"Absolutely not."

"Does morbidity mean side effects?"

"Yes."

"I believe my anal sphincter has become quite tight; my feces are still stringy."

"Your rectum is probably still inflamed and swollen. I doubt it's your sphincter. Well, let's see what we find."

Donning latex gloves, he gave me a digital, which was surprisingly painful.

"It's not your sphincter," he said. "Great! The nodule's much smaller. I'd say by 75 percent. Your rectum *is* inflamed."

Withdrawing his finger, removing the gloves and washing his hands, he said, "I'd like you to use hydrocortisone suppositories twice a day for a week."

"We're doing okay?"

"Much better than that. We're doing fine!"

JULY 17, 1993. So my PSA is now 8.9. Or rather, that's what it was on July 6. That's excellent, as Dr. North said. But 8.9 was only a month after therapy. What will the number be three months from July 6? And three months after that? And a year after therapy? I wonder what my cancer cells are up to these days. What do they have planned for me? In short, I've savored my good news the past several days, but now, occasionally, I find myself wondering about its true goodness. After all, 8.9 isn't so small a figure. I ask myself, why wasn't the number 6, or even 5? And what about John Darrough, whose cancer recurred after radiation? And Morton Blumberg, whose cancer also recurred, and who's apparently in much worse shape than Darrough?

At lunch today my friend John Lowrance told me a joke. An elderly man is sitting on a park bench. A frog hops over to him and says, "Kiss me and I'll turn into a beautiful woman."

"What's that you said?" asks the man, staring at the frog.

"Kiss me and I'll turn into a beautiful woman."

The man picks the frog up and puts it into his pocket.

The frog says, "Didn't you hear me? I said, 'Kiss me and I'll turn into a beautiful woman.'"

The man says, "At my age I'd rather have a talking frog."

Nine

July 22 to August 16, 1993

JULY 22, 1993. After showering this morning I happened to glance at my abdomen, as a consequence of which I wrote two jingles.

Where, oh where, is my pubic hair?
I wonder what I've done wrong.
It frankly was beyond compare,
And now I've only a song.

And:

X rays! X rays!
Murder's being done!
Not in the cathedral,
But under the hospital sun.
Cancer, Cancer,
Fly away now.
My prostate's in a pickle.
High tech will show you how.

I interviewed Harry Stengel, our support group leader, this afternoon in the large living room of his spacious, ranch-style King City house surrounded by gardens. He was aware that I was writing a book about my prostate cancer, and that I hoped to broaden its scope by interviewing a number of fellow prostate cancerites (to coin a word). Throughout the interview I was aware of an odor of wild roses so strong that at times it threatened to distract me. His voice was soft, gentle, as was his whole manner. He had a good, cultivated mind. White hair; a roundish, kindly face; a sensitive mouth; friendly blue eyes. He probably thought he could lose some weight; but he carried his weight well.

I had become very fond of him in the three months since I had met him. He was a superb, outgoing, caring leader of the group, taking careful notes during the meetings; sending the members a report on each meeting; notifying them of interesting developments in prostate cancer research, or of coming events; and so on. He was so much the soul of the successful group that I sometimes wondered if the group could survive his leaving it.

In 1989 [he began], *when I had a routine physical, the doctor said my PSA was up just a bit, something under 10, but not to worry. Next year my physical showed that my PSA was up to 59, so he said, "Well, we'd better do something about this," and sent me to a urologist. This was in May. I hadn't been very conscious of prostate cancer. Instead, I had been worried about lung cancer, because until I was about fifty I smoked. My brother, who was a heavy smoker, had died of lung cancer. I don't know if he had prostate cancer too. The urologist did the finger test, and there was this ill-defined lump, which is bad to begin with. He did an ultrasound, then took four specimens in a needle biopsy. The biopsy came back positive, so he sent me off to get a CAT scan and a bone scan. The bone scan was positive. There were five or six lesions.*

By this time I felt just awful. I was completely unprepared for my mortality. I hadn't thought about it even though my father had died of prostate cancer. I was in good health and I had never had any physical problems, so my cancer came as a terrible blow. What was most traumatic was this harrowing sense of loneliness. I have a great wife and four great kids, who all rallied around the flag; but you know, there was nobody I could really share my feelings with. And it

146

was this, more than anything else, that I had trouble coping with. In the past, in difficult times, I had always turned to the family. Turned to my wife. She was always there, she could always understand. But this. . . . There was something about this. . . . Here I was, way out in left field, and everybody else was out there, and I had no idea what the hell I was doing. This was the worst thing I had to cope with personally. It took a hell of a long time. I don't suppose I made my peace with myself until maybe a year later.

My urologist told me I had a year and a half to live, or maybe a little more, maybe four or five if I were lucky. I went down to this chief of gynecology—gynecology!—I mean oncology—at Georgetown University. Ugh! He couldn't have been more unsympathetic. His manner was really clinical.

"How long ago were you given a year and a half?" I asked.

It's now three years.

"Do you remember your Gleason number?"

It was 4 plus 4. Some people say 8 is low. Others say it's high. Some doctors over at Fox-Chase said, "Gee, what are you worried about? It could be so much worse." But if it's 8, and 10's the highest, it can't get much worse, right? My PSA went down to 0.5 within two months after I got on Lupron and Eulexin, and it's been there ever since. My urologist put me on Lupron and Eulexin, but on only three Eulexin pills a day, which surprised the oncologist at Georgetown, because he wondered why he didn't put me on six a day. You take the Eulexin every eight hours, around the clock.

"The Lupron is an injection?"

Yes.

"Your PSA is wonderful!"

It is, it is! And so, about a year and a half ago, and my PSA still being down there, I began to come to terms with my cancer, to recognize I wasn't about to depart immediately. It was about that time my sense of loneliness began to recede. Also, about that time I started organizing the support group, and that was a real boost for me, because for the first time I felt I could talk to people who really understood what the hell I was up against. The first two or three sessions we had, all of us talked about our own situations, and it was then I really began to come out of my isolation.

I did a lot of reading of books around then. I read Max Lerner's book Wrestling with the Angel, *and I found him a little too glib, maybe. He had lymphoma, and then prostate cancer, yet he lived for twelve years, I think. You know, everybody would look at me who knew I had cancer, as if, "God, Harry, Jesus it's tough, it's tough."* [Harry Stengel laughed.] *"But how come you look so good?" Max Lerner experienced this too. He said people would say, "Gee, Max, you look great." And he was the one who responded by saying, "Well, I look better than I feel. And I feel better than I am."*

Anyhow, I had a lot of intestinal distress, presumably from the Eulexin. I guess 10 percent of people, it affects them negatively. Flatulence, diarrhea. I was feeling miserable. They tried all sorts of things to stop the diarrhea, because I was running maybe four or five times a day. And that still isn't gone, although it's much better. I get it maybe once a month. They say it's the lactose base of the Eulexin that affects some people. And yet I never had trouble with milk.

"Did you have bone pain?"

No. I have a little pain up here [feeling his upper rib under his left arm]. *There's one lesion that doesn't want to go away. The others disappeared. It isn't constant. I don't know if it's my imagination or not. The first year I had a bone scan every six months. Now I have one once a year.*

"The lesions disappeared?"

All except this one. And I guess there's another one over here [feeling his right side]. *But anyway, they don't bother me.*

"Do you keep getting ultrasounds?"

No, because the prostate has shrunk to almost nothing.

"Because of the Lupron and Eulexin?"

Yes.

"How did this thing go that far in one year, with a PSA of 59?"

Nobody knows. I have a feeling, Charles, that my physician, because of my father's history of prostate cancer . . . I think he goofed. That first year, when the thing was up a bit, he said, "Oh well, Harry,

not ready I walk out. I tell them, "My time is as valuable as his." I
wear a chip on my shoulder. My wife says, "But Harry, you're sick.
You need them." Since this all got started, I've become crotchety, dif-
ficult, emotional.

JULY 27, 1993, CAPE MAY POINT, NEW JERSEY. I'm visiting Cousin
Erik and Molly here for several days. I've come not only because I love them and enjoy being with them, but also because
I'm going to interview Erik about his experience with the radical prostatectomy. The rented, rambling, all-year, jerrybuilt
house is built on stilts as insurance against ocean floods and
heaps of sand. Erik is a large, charming, highly literate and articulate man who can be very funny when he's in the right
mood. He's a collector of all kinds of odds and ends: ancient
hand tools, cookie jars, baseball bats, chandeliers, ad infinitum. He and Molly, a large woman who's an inveterate reader,
are a congenial pair. After all these years of marriage she still
laughs heartily, sometimes to the point of tears, at his jokes;
and tolerates his collection mania.

Summer heat; oceanic, southern New Jersey humidity; scrub
trees; the grittiness of sand underfoot; sounds of the pounding
surf; mosquitoes at night the size of condors; a great variety of
migratory birds and birders; summer socializing: Erik and
Molly's children and grandchildren, and a pleasant chaos of
chatter and eating; sand castles; surf play; beach umbrellas; early
mornings; long evenings.

On the morning of the 25th and 26th here I did my usual
three-mile fast walk, and yesterday, in addition, I put in at least
two more miles walking around Cape May. On Lincoln Road I
stay on the two yellow lines in the middle because the road is
most horizontal there and because there's no traffic at so early an
hour (7:30 A.M.).

Today an elderly man, coming up behind me on a very
old bike, said, "Good morning." We were near the end of the

road where the nuns hang out. I wondered if he was connected with them.

"Good morning," I replied.

"You look as if you're doing the sobriety test," he said, giving me a belly laugh.

I interviewed Erik this afternoon when we were alone in the house. The others had gone to the beach or to play tennis.

In September of '91, I think it was [he said], *I had a free prostate exam during Prostate Cancer Awareness Week. A youngish doctor, having done a digital on me, said in a matter-of-fact voice, "I don't like what I feel. I'm a urologist. Come to my office in Tarrytown and I'll do a biopsy." He gave me his name. "What about a sonogram?" I asked. Getting the impression he didn't have an ultrasound machine, I decided to find someone else.*

The second urologist, Dr. Fledermaus, did a digital and said, "I have to compliment the young doctor. If I were tired I might miss feeling this lump. It's very small, and high up. Because of its position I doubt it's cancer, but we'll do a sonogram and a biopsy to make sure." My PSA was 4.2. He called a couple of days later, said the biopsy was positive, and wanted to meet with me and Molly to discuss what to do.

When we went to see him he said, "We can do nothing. Or we can do radiation, which isn't a cure. Or we can remove the prostate. A prostatectomy is the only real cure. Now, you should know that right after a prostatectomy you may feel as if a truck had hit you. And both radiation and a prostatectomy may make you impotent or incontinent, possibly permanently. But these are rare possibilities, and if they happen, we have ways of dealing with them. Look, you can live into your eighties. You're in good physical condition. You're a perfect candidate for a prostatectomy. Think about it and decide what you want to do."

"Would you do the operation?"

"Yes."

"Will I need blood?"

152

"Yes."

"Can I provide my own?"

"Yes. On a schedule at the hospital. A unit a week. Five units."

"Did he ever mention the ten-year or fifteen-year survival rate of radiation as against prostatectomy?" I asked.

All he said was that a prostatectomy is permanent and is the only cure for prostate cancer.

I said, "My cousin Murray has prostate cancer. He was told there are different degrees of such cancer."

Dr. Fledermaus said bluntly, "Cancer is cancer."

Molly and I went home, discussed it, and I said, "If it's okay with you, I elect to have it out."

"Did he mention a Gleason number?" I asked. "Or the fact that some of the cancer cells may be very aggressive, whereas others may be very timid? Did you get a copy of the biopsy report?"

I saw nothing. He was very definite about cancer being cancer.

"Did you consider getting a second opinion?"

As far as I was concerned, I had had one. The young urologist was the one who had found the lump, and Dr. Fledermaus had corroborated him. Dr. Fledermaus seemed to have good credentials, and we had good rapport. There are limits to how many opinions you can get. He didn't make light of my cancer. He did mention you can die due to the general anesthesia or the operation, but said it's unlikely. When Molly and I returned and said we had decided to have the prostate out, he said, "That's what I would have done."

I said, "Look, I'm sexually active, and you say I'm in great shape. I want you to be very, very careful not to sever any of the nerves which will affect my ability to get an erection."

He said, "In your case I'll be very careful," and we laughed.

He said I needed a private general physician to see me in the hospital. I asked him to recommend someone, and he did. He said he would remove the lymph nodes, and if they showed cancer, that would be the end of the operation, he would sew me up.

I had a pre-op workup: CAT scan, bone scan, various physical tests. One of the nurses said the hospital would provide me with a morphine machine, and I could get a supply of morphine by pushing a button. I wouldn't be able to get it beyond a certain point, but she thought I should have one.

So Molly and I drove to the hospital early one December morning. I was in good spirits. Dr. Scott, a young man, came around and introduced himself. Around noon I was wheeled in for the operation. The next thing I knew, I woke up in the recovery room, and Molly was there. The painkillers were still working. Later I started to tap away at the morphine, which came through an IV.

A friend of mine had said to me, "Tell your wife that if you start acting strange, it's the morphine. Some people are allergic to it."

I remember my son, Bruce, and his wife, Lynn, coming into my room with one of those aluminum balloons.

I said, "Get that out of here. I don't want things floating near the ceiling."

It took me a day or so to realize I had an allergy to the morphine. I made the nurses take the machine away. And I insisted on being put into a reclining chair, because I felt I was choking while lying on my back in the bed.

Dr. Fledermaus said to me, "The next couple of days are crucial in terms of avoiding pneumonia. You must keep your lungs clear. And you've got to get out of bed soon and start walking. The more walking you do, the faster you'll get out of here."

They gave me something to blow on. Your abdomen hurts, yet you have to blow and blow. I was afraid the catheter might come loose. I learned later it's anchored with an internal balloon. The first couple of nights I slept in a reclining chair, with my feet on an ottoman. Once, Dr. Fledermaus came in at midnight while I had my feet briefly off the ottoman.

He said, "You're looking for blood clots. Keep your feet up."

I forgot you can wind the hospital bed all the way up, almost to a sitting position, so I suffered unnecessarily trying to sleep in the chair. I think it was the morphine.

In spite of the pain, I began walking up and down the corridor, with the catheter tied to the IV pole. After a couple of days I felt I was bearing the whole weight of the catheter. I couldn't understand it, because the catheter was being held up by the pole. Then, with alarm, I sensed a tremendous weight between my legs. I gingerly felt under my gown. My scrotum was about the size of a grapefruit. When I mentioned this to Dr. Fledermaus, he said it was fairly normal, because he had removed the lymph nodes, and the fluid had to go somewhere, and I was lucky it hadn't gone to my chest, which would have been more painful.

I continued my walking. To my horror, my scrotum blew up to the size of a volley ball. It was hard to walk, because I was dragging this huge thing between my legs. I mentioned this to Dr. Fledermaus and said, "I think I should have a suspensory." He ordered one, but it turned out to be for a normal scrotum.

I asked, "How long will this last?"

He said, "It will probably take about six months for it to recover."

I said to myself, "I can't live with this thing for that long."

While walking, my thighs and crotch would get chafed. I felt as if I had elephantiasis. But fortunately my scrotum pretty much returned to normal in three or four weeks.

One afternoon an elderly priest walked into my room and said, "If there's anything I can do for you, prayers or the like, please let me know."

I said, "I happen to be of the Jewish faith, although basically I'm an atheist."

He said, "Do you mind if I rest with you for a while?"

Sitting down, he said prostate problems are one of the occupational hazards of being a priest.

Another visitor was a beautiful female rabbi from a nearby temple. When she heard I was under the same religious umbrella, she chatted with me a bit.

While being driven home I felt a terrific pain in my right arm, mainly in my wrist, and I said to myself, "This has to be the result of all the difficulty the nurses had in finding the veins for the shunt." I was weak, and needed help getting out of the car and into my house.

The first two weeks at home I slept downstairs though my bedroom is upstairs. I was depressed, weak and incontinent. I went to see an orthopedic surgeon about the pain in my arm. It turned out, after a neurological exam, that damage had already been done to certain nerves, and that the sooner I had the ulnar nerve moved, the better off I'd be. I was back in the hospital in March, again with general anesthesia.

After a while I no longer had to wear diapers, but at night I still used a rubber mat in bed. I knew I wasn't voiding all my urine, so I told Dr. Fledermaus, "I'm having a lot of trouble urinating."

He said, "Don't worry about it. It'll take care of itself."

Finally, I called him and said, "Look, I've got to see you. I've developed hemorrhoids from squeezing so much to get the urine out."

He said, "You'd better come in."

When he catheterized me he took one look and said, "We have to do this in the hospital, and pretty soon. Your urethra has developed scar tissue. As you told me yourself, you have a tendency to keloids."

So I was back in the hospital in July. I had called another surgeon and said, "After I have my urethra reamed out and while I'm still on the operating table, will you remove my hemorrhoids?"

This time I had a local, thank goodness. They wanted to give me Tylenol with codeine for the pain, but the pain was so great I said, "You have to give me Demerol." They told me I couldn't have it more than once every three hours.

After the first day, Dr. Fledermaus said, "You're ready to go home."

I said, "No way. I'm in too much pain."

He said, "Well, we'll have to put this extra day on the general surgeon's account, because as far as I'm concerned you're ready to leave."

I left the hospital after two days. On my next important visit to him he said he would have to catheterize me again. He put the tube in, then a funnel into the tube, and kept pouring more and more water into the funnel to fill the bladder. Then he corked the tube. To my delight, the water pressure blew the cork, and he got a full shower.

My PSA has remained at 0.00, which indicates, at least so far, that none of the cancer cells escaped. The incontinence lasted about a year. It would stop for a while, then come back. I'm almost 100 percent recovered now. I think the effects of the incontinence were more mental than physical. Once, Molly wanted me to go to the theater with her, saying I could wear a diaper. I said I wouldn't be comfortable watching a play and urinating at the same time. I was depressed. I didn't talk much.

Regarding my impotence, Dr. Fledermaus said, "Sometimes it takes about a year before you function sexually. If you don't function after a year and a half, we'll do something about it."

I said, "What happened during the operation?"

He said, "Unfortunately I had to cut one of the nerves which control erection."

A year and a half after the operation, he recommended the vacuum system and I bought it from him. I've been unable to use it for intercourse. Yes, you do get a large erection, but the penis doesn't seem to be sensitive. And I found, while practicing with the device, that the rubber band that acts as a tourniquet at the base of the penis to hold the blood in the organ is so painful that it would probably take much of the pleasure out of sex. The rubber bands are the great problem with that system. The company gives you four bands of varying pressure. A large penis would require the weakest band. If necessary, you use two bands to maintain an erection. I found that even with the two toughest bands my erection wasn't maintained. Also, aside from the pain, my penis, instead of being like the trunk of a tree, flaps in the wind. It's erect, but not stiff. I imagine it would be difficult to penetrate with it.

Another method is the injection system. To interrupt foreplay to jab yourself with a needle at the base of the penis doesn't strike me as being fun. A third method, the silicone implant, which a friend of mine uses and which he raves about, requires general anesthesia and a stay in the hospital for two or three days. I haven't been able to have an orgasm since the operation, and I suspect I'm incapable of having one.

"Does Molly have any feeling about the fact that sex has ended for her?" I asked.

She feels that our spiritual relationship is more important than sex. It would be nice to have sex. However, it's not the most important thing in our lives at our age. I still haven't made my peace with the lack of

sex. If I had it to do over again, for the sake of sex I might opt for radi-
ation, although I realize that impotence is a possible side effect of radi-
ation. But now that it's over, the lack of sex doesn't bother me as much
as it did some time ago.

AUGUST 3, 1993. When I spoke by phone with Dr. North this morning, I sang the pubic hair jingle for him. He laughed and said, "The two of us should go on the road with a doctor-and-patient routine about prostate cancer."

I had told golden-haired Marie Izant that I wanted to interview her for my book about my prostate cancer, and she had agreed, and so we met in the lobby of the Oncology Center at 1:00 today and we walked to a nearby pizza restaurant. She was in whites. During lunch I learned she's leaving the Oncology Center on the 20th and will begin working as a radiation therapy technician at a medical center in Oldtown, New Jersey, on the 23rd. If I had received this news in the midst of my therapy I would have been upset. I had always enjoyed her warmth, candor and infectious laughter, and her presence had come to feel like an essential part of my healing process.

"Why are you leaving?" I asked.

"I got complaints from patients. I'm too outspoken. Remember I said you danced?"

"I did dance, and I liked your noticing it. What you call outspoken I call your irony. Your mentioning it that way, and laughing about it, made me feel closer to you. That feeling of closeness between me and the techs and nurses and Dr. North was very healing."

"That 'irony' is what other patients didn't like. I used to work in a hospital in Trenton. The patients there were less affluent than in King City, and more appreciative. King City patients tend to be touchy, demanding, difficult, at least in my experience. One woman asked me where I was born. I said Trenton. She said, 'Oh, so you're a peasant.'"

"Was she kidding?"

"No. Some patients get angry when we're even a little late, as if we're fooling around. One woman was furious because we were ten minutes late. She said, 'What do you girls do in there? Goof off while you keep me waiting?' We tried to explain, but she wouldn't listen. Some patients are angry about their sickness, and they take it out on us."

"Will you get more money on your new job?"

"A little. But I'll have a much longer commute."

"Do you ever wonder if *you* have cancer?"

"Usually not. But once, I thought there was a little lump in the right side of my throat. I went to see a doctor. It was nothing."

"What's the hardest job you've had to do with patients?"

"Handling a young man's testicle. We sometimes get a patient in his twenties who has testicular cancer. Usually one testicle has been removed. The other has to be protected against radiation as we irradiate his pelvic area. We put a block under the testicle, then cover the testicle with a shield. We don't like to do that, so sometimes we teach the patient how to prepare his testicle himself, and we check that it's done right. We have a high cure rate for testicular cancer."

"Does his penis get irradiated?"

"We turn it to one side so it avoids the radiation."

"Has a patient ever had an erection while being treated?"

"Not in my experience. But I heard somebody say they did see it once or twice. It's nothing. It's part of the job."

"Do patients ever make passes?"

"No. When I worked in Trenton we sometimes had prisoners come in to be treated, but even they were well behaved. We usually get used to almost everything, but occasionally something upsets me, like a young woman whose breast cancer has spread to her brain, and we're irradiating her brain, and we know she may not make it, and she has a six-year-old daughter. That's hard."

"There was a very sad woman in the waiting room a couple of times when I was there. Do you remember her?"

"She made a fuss about having to expose her breasts. She was being treated for breast cancer. Our patients are on camera. That's necessary. We need to keep in touch with them when we're outside the treatment room. One day she noticed the monitor and made a terrible fuss. She said strangers passing by could see her. We assured her no strangers were ever allowed in that area."

"Are your parents alive?"

"My mom had breast cancer. After a while she complained about pains in her back. She went to a chiropractor, who said she needed spinal adjustments and he could help her. He treated her, but the pains continued, so she saw a medical doctor. The doctor did some tests and detected jaundice. She died two weeks later."

"Liver cancer? The breast cancer had metastasized?"

"Yes."

"How old was she?"

"In her mid-fifties."

"What about your father?"

"He's ornery."

"What do you mean?"

"Just that."

She laughed. I had a renewed sense of her warm, vibrant personality.

AUGUST 16, 1993. When I reported to my urologist's office at 1:15, a nurse led me to an exam room and handed me a stainless steel pan. After she left I voided. Entering, Dr. Gilroy, looking fit and wearing a white coat, a vividly green-striped shirt and a green tie, asked me to sit on a gurney.

"Some questions for you," he said. "Appetite?"

"Good."

"Weight?"

"Down a bit."

"Energy?"

"I normally walk three miles daily at about four miles an hour. I used to do it in forty-four or forty-five minutes. Lately I've done it in forty-two. A couple of times at forty-one, forty."

"Stools. Any pain?"

"No."

"Difficulty voiding?"

"No."

"Any blood?"

"No."

"Urination. Pain?"

"No."

"Blood?"

"No."

"Difficulty voiding?"

"No."

"Any dribbling?"

"No."

"No little drops?"

"None."

"How's the stream?"

"Good. Especially if I drink a lot of fluid."

He had me lower my trousers and undershorts and lie on my back. He examined my penis, checking the opening, then my testicles, occasionally squeezing one gently. The squeezing was slightly unpleasant. He palpated my abdominal and pelvic areas. Asking me to sit up, he squeezed and/or punched various parts of my back, spine and ribs, always asking, "Any pain? Any pain here?" He was checking for evidence of prostatic bone cancer. There was no pain of recent origin.

"Stand up and bend over, with your elbows on the end of the table," he said.

The digital was more prolonged and painful than I expected. When would he stop? Why was he being so thorough? Why did this one hurt more than Dr. North's? Wiping my behind with some soft tissue, he said, "Come to my office when you're ready."

"What did you feel? A change in the tumor?" I asked when I joined him.

"It's smaller. Also the gland. I won't be surprised if the gland gets still smaller. There are a few pus cells in your urine but it's nothing to be concerned about. It's to be expected, since you had radiation cystitis. It takes a while for it to clear up. You're in good shape. A PSA of 8.9 a month after radiation is an excellent sign. If the PSA goes down to 4 or lower, we think that's probably a cure. If it doesn't, we wonder about the possibility of recurrence. It's not only the PSA we look at. It's the PSA curve, the direction in which it's going."

"But if I don't go down to 4, what about the fact that you called my gland a monster gland?"

"That's right. We need to take that into consideration. There's something called a PSA density, the proportion of the PSA to the size of the gland. It's two and a half months since you finished therapy. Ten months from now we should have a pretty good idea of where you stand. Of what's a normal PSA for you. A cancer-free PSA. Until then we'll check your PSA every three months. If it's stable a year after therapy, I'll see you twice a year."

"My acid phosphatase is 3.9. I saw Dr. Daniel Redmont recently to report on my condition. He said he doesn't pay attention to acid phosphatase anymore."

"I don't either. Some urologists, like myself, don't even order it. PSA's the thing we watch."

As we went to his office manager's office, where I would pay for the visit, he put his arm around me. I responded in kind.

Ten

August 17 to September 22, 1993

AUGUST 17, 1993. This afternoon I interviewed John Darrough of the prostate cancer support group in his very quiet house in Plainsboro, New Jersey. My reason for selecting him is that his cancer recurred several years after radiation therapy, something of particular importance to me because I too had had radiation. Also, because of his articulateness at the group meetings, I sensed he was a good subject for an interview.

He's the member who always attends meetings with his wife, Barbara. I like them both. They're outgoing, friendly and intelligent. Like Harry Stengel and Erik, they know I'm writing a book about my prostate cancer. Darrough looks very fit. Both his words and his actions tend to be intense and rapid. His speech pattern at times sounded new and interesting to me, and almost a little foreign. I neglected to ask him what might account for it.

He sat on a sofa during the interview, facing me across a coffee table. I sat on a chair. Barbara occupied an armchair on his left and somewhat apart from him. Though in the beginning she acknowledged by her silence and body language that the interview belonged to him, she later, at my invitation, joined the discussion.

I figure to myself [he began], *"Yeah, I have an affliction. It's there, and it's something I'll have to live with for as long as I go." I was fifty-nine when I first had the necessity for a transurethral resection of the* prostate. I went to a urologist because I was having trouble urinating. He says, "There's a good reason for it. A swelling is blocking your urethra. I'm going to do a section on you."

I said, "Fine, but what does it entail?"

He says, "I'll knock you out, then I'll go into the penis, ream out the material in the prostate, and cleanse the gland."

I didn't realize I was going to have a catheter in me for five or six days. That catheter was a shock. That is an experience I don't like to ask anybody to go through, for the simple reason that I spasmed in the area of my bladder. My body wanted to reject it, and so I would get these terrible cramps—constantly. Very difficult. Sometimes I'd get it during the night, and there'd be nobody to answer me. The morning nurse would come on and say, "What have you been doing?"

I'd say, "I haven't been sleeping, that's one thing."

Well, in about five days or six days they removed the catheter, and it was one of the greatest reliefs in my entire life. Then, when I was released from the hospital, I was told to use a large diaper. I asked the doctor about the biopsy.

He says, "There's no cancerous tissue, but I see what looks like a precancerous condition."

I said, "What are you going to do about it?"

He says, "I'm giving this information by letter to your internist, who should follow up on you every six months to a year."

I was age fifty-nine then. I did not return to the internist until I was age sixty-two. Nobody gave me any warning to come in and have this thing checked. I went in for other things, but nobody ever checked the prostate. Now then. This happens too, I think, by the grace of God. I'm employed by the RCA laboratories here, and RCA sells out to General Electric. I'm sixty-two, and all from sixty on up are given retirement packages. In order for me to collect a lump sum, I have to pass a complete physical. So off I go to my internist, who happens to be a different one. The other one retired. Also the urologist retired.

So this internist looks at my records and says, "It says here you should have been monitored. I'm going to examine you. I'll write you *up as okay, but you go to the urologist as fast as you can, because I detect something here."*

So I go home and tell Barb and make a quick appointment with Dr. Dickens. Dr. Dickens says, "Oh yes, there's something suspicious here. And I wonder if you would be willing to do something."

I said, "What is that?"

He said, "We have new ultrasound equipment. We have never used it, and I am going to be the first to test it, and if you're willing, I'll test it on you at no cost."

Oh boy. That's expensive stuff. So I said, "Fine, doctor."

He said, "At the same time, I'm going to biopsy you."

So I went through this. The biopsy was positive. From age sixty-two to sixty-five Dr. Dickens did six ultrascans, and he had a record of the actual growth, if any, in that area. And for me there was none. He offered me two options.

He said, "I can surgically remove."

I said, "What will the aftereffects be?"

He says (he was quite open about this), "You run the possibility of being incontinent and impotent. You have another option. Seeing a radiation oncologist. See him. See what's there."

So I went to Dr. Mapleton and he goes over me. And I said, "What would be this procedure? And what would be my prognosis after this?"

He says, "As far as any of that other stuff goes, there's nothing to worry about here, radiation. Nothing invasive. No incontinence. No this, no that. No anything."

I said, "Hey, I'm taking this." I was that kind of person.

So Mapleton goes through the procedure. You know, they stuff all that stuff in you and work your whole body up. And that to me was the worst part of the entire procedure. The radiation—that's like nothing. I go there and lie on the table and the machine goes around me and I'm in there maybe three, four minutes a day for eight weeks, with the exception of Saturdays and Sundays. For a total of about 6000 rads. About thirty-five treatments. I had some minor effects. Radiation burns in my rectal area and around the penis. I lost all my pubic and rectum hair. Mild burns. They weren't bad.

"What was your PSA before you started?" I asked.

In the beginning, 4 to 8. I'm sixty-eight now. After the radiation it was 10. It went down, then up, and remained at that level for about five and a half years. Six months ago Dr. Lerocki got suspicious because it was rising, so he had me come in every month for a complete checkup and internal. Plus PSA. He did another biopsy. He took five specimens. It was positive—on one side. It's a terrible procedure. For God's sake, I'm lying there with tears in my eyes. He says, "All right now, get ready."

Bam!

Dr. Lerocki says, "Look, this is isolated. I want another opinion. I'm sending you to Memorial in New York with all your data."

"That's when we read it," said Barbara Darrough, who was present at the interview.

That's when I came to see some of the stuff that was written, and I said to myself, "Jesus, what the hell is this?" I go to Memorial, and the two doctors—one, he gave me everything you get. They took blood from the word go. Finally the head physician comes in and says, "There's no involvement of the seminal vesicles. It's still encapsulated in the gland. How'd you like to get rid of this completely for the rest of your life? You're a good candidate for cryosurgery at Allegheny Hospital in Pittsburgh."

So I looked into Allegheny and found it would require me to go in and out of there five different times. Surgical cost, $13,000. Approximate hospital and other costs, another $7,000.

I said, "Fine. Now what's the coverage?" Nobody would cover it. Medicare wouldn't. Nobody. Experimental. So, I did not get it. I can't put out $20,000. I says, "Look, candidate or not, unless somebody promises to pay some of these costs," I says, "no way."

This business of having it removed for life is for the birds. Removed for life? One guy, two years, it's back again. Another guy, two and a half years, back again. And there's a chance of impotence. Also, that it will return over a period of six months to a year after the procedure. You see, you don't get these verbals.

He tells you, "Man, this is great! You're going to be free for the rest of your life!" But I would have been in another experiment. In the second two hundred men. So I went back to Lerocki.

Lerocki says, "Hey, they gave you a good report. You don't have anything anywhere except where it is now. The only thing I want to do is monitor you. We'll determine month to month how we go with this. I'm going to give you a complete physical plus the internal plus the blood work every month. Every six months, though, you must have an MRI and a bone scan and a chest X ray. The reason for this is because many times, if you just have a urologist, he'll concentrate only on your affliction. Yet there may be something else going on in your body. I want to cover the entire picture."

I said, "Okay. Fine."

So he's been doing this. And my last PSA was 20. It hovers. It's 16 to 20. According to him, this is within experimental error, the way tests are run. He says, "This small change that exists here, I don't regard it as significant. If we hit something that starts showing up, a rapid increase, I got medication. But I don't want to give it to you yet." This was the end of June. He says, "Take the summer off. Don't come back to me until September."

I mean, he goes over everything. So I'm letting it go.

And he has begun to deal with my head.

He says, "You know, you've been handling this thing almost six years now." He says, "You know it's there." And he says, "You're holding pretty well with everything." He says, "But I want to talk to you about your mind." He says, "Any time you're depressed or you feel you're bothered by this thing, tell me." He's taking all ends of this. I'm very appreciative. I'm very happy with that man. And Barb was brought in to every one of my checkups. She has to be brought in for her opinion. And I think it's great.

"Another thing you have to take into consideration when you think about therapy or drugs is, are you sexually active?" said Barbara Darrough. "If you're not, there's no worry there. At the time we found out John had cancer, we had my mother living with us. She was eighty-eight. She had been with us a couple of years. We also learned she had lung cancer. It was terrible. She wasn't a smoker. My father was a smoker, though. The lung goes to the brain. They worried about that with her. She had colon cancer when she was seventy, but everything was all right. This was not a secondary cancer. This was another kind."

While I was being treated I was taking her for her treatments. We kept my treatments away from her knowledge until she was completely through with hers and I was completely through with mine. When it was all done, we let her know I had problems too. I started radiation in March and finished in June.

"Any side effects?" I asked.

The thing is, I'm a strange person. When something like diarrhea happens, I just say, "Okay, that's part of it," and I go along with it. It may be severe, and I don't know, because I'm accepting it.

"But you did have that accident," said Barbara Darrough.

Oh God. I swear to God, that was embarrassing. I'm driving in my car from the garage. I'm on my way home here. And I lose control. Completely. I can't wait to get into the house. I was so embarrassed. Fortunately no one was home then. But they had told me that was a possibility. I accepted it. But it didn't mean I wasn't embarrassed. And I was angry about having done such a thing.

"John usually is in control," said Barbara Darrough. "That's why he doesn't like surgery."

"Did Mapleton ever talk about the recurrence rate after radiation?" I asked.

He said, "Oh, you have no problem with this." I was told that by Mapleton and by Dickens. I would die of something else, not prostate cancer.

"What was your Gleason number?"

3 or 4. I had one in the beginning that was 2 to 3. 3 to 4 was after the radiation. In reference to my brother, for God's sake, they took everything out of that kid. He didn't know what hit him until maybe five years later, when he suddenly realized. But I lost him only . . . what? . . . eight months ago? Heart attack. He was sixty-five. He was in his early fifties when they did the prostatectomy on him. It scared the hell out of my older brother and me, because after the operation this doctor tells us, "You know, I think your brother is cancerous."

We said, "What?"

He says, "I'll have to wait to be absolutely certain. I'm getting the tissue checked."

So we came back three or four days later and he says, "It was negative. No problem."

But, you know, we were struck with this thing.

"Years ago the doctors were God," said Barbara Darrough. "Put on a pedestal. They gave you no information. I don't like the idea that John's angry. He *is* angry. I remember telling Dr. Dickens about it. Angry because the cancer returned. Dr. Dickens hemmed and hawed. I asked him if there was any therapy, any support group. I was so upset. John was calmer about it."

That's how we joined the support group. That's why she comes with me all the time.

"We have a daughter who's a social worker," said Barbara Darrough. "In fact, the summer when both John and my mother heard the news that they had cancer, I went the whole summer to counseling (I'm a teacher, I had the summer off), because I just couldn't take it. Here are these two people upon whom I depended (my mother all my life; a very dominant woman), and my husband is a strong husband figure. Both had a fatal disease. I was so distraught, I just couldn't take it. My mother, who didn't know what was wrong, kept saying to me—. You know the old saw about you're lazy if you sleep late. I was still teaching then. John was retired, and he slept until 10 or 11 in the morning. He was so fatigued. His door was always closed."

Later, when we explained it to her, it was okay.

"Most impotent men, I gather, say the lack of sex doesn't bother their mates," I remarked.

"You know, maybe a man can make an effort," said Barbara Darrough. "Even though he can't have an orgasm, why doesn't he try to have her get one?"

You know, the thing that bothered me, in the prelude to the actual radiation, was the mapping. I had to go three days to be mapped. After the third day Dr. Mapleton says, "You got a lot of stuff in your system. Drink a lot of liquid, and it'll pass."

Well, it didn't. I'm the kind of a guy who goes to the bathroom every morning like clockwork. Aw! Three days I didn't move! Aw! It was terrible!

"We were at church," said Barbara Darrough, "and he was having trouble. It was Saturday night. We were having mass. And he said to me, 'I can't stay here anymore.' We went back to the house, and he got rid of it, and he stuffed up the plumbing."

I had to clear the whole thing by hand. I didn't know this was going to happen. He said, "It'll pass." It passed, all right.

I went to Aptos, California, a village some ten or fifteen miles south of Santa Cruz, the day after interviewing Darrough, and almost immediately received an emotional shock that reduced me to tears. Upon ringing the house doorbell of Peter and Penelope Kenez, good friends of mine whom I was going to visit for several days and then housesit for for a month while they went to Russia and Hungary, I was surprised not to be greeted by the bass barking of my dear friend Matsko, a female German shepherd. (Matsko is a Hungarian name.) When Peter opened the door, I asked, "Why no barking?"

"Matsko is dying. He's in the kitchen," Peter informed me quietly.

Peter, a professor of Soviet history at the University of California at Santa Cruz, originally from Hungary, never failed to refer to Matsko as *he*. There are lovable linguistic rationalizations for this that aren't worth going into at the moment. Peter knew as well as Matsko the difference between a female dog and a male one; yet in the case of Matsko, a "Hungarian" German shepherd, he would blithely say, on occasion, "He's in heat."

Following him into the kitchen, I saw Matsko stretched out on the floor, breathing heavily, eyes glazed. Though I called her name, she gave no sign of recognizing me. Twice she made a hopeless effort to stand.

I loved her. She and I had lived alone together in the Kenez house the previous summer; but I had known her long before then. But that summer we had taken hikes in the Forest of Nisene Marks State Park nearby, which contained the epicenter of the tragic earthquake of October 1989; and we had descended steep, sometimes stony trails; and on turning back toward home (she was leashed), without my asking her to she had hauled me up those trails with such speed that I had felt I was effortlessly flying. I was convinced (and still am) she was doing this to spare me because of my advanced age. And because she knew I loved her. And because she loved me.

Peter now explained that Matsko had gotten increasingly tired and unsteady on her legs during the past couple of weeks; that only yesterday a female vet had said she had inoperable cancer; and that the vet was coming at 6:00 to give her a lethal injection and take her away. And so, without any warning I was about to lose an important friend whom I had assumed was in perfect health and who would joyously share the house with me. And I was still fairly fresh from radiation therapy; also, I could feel the little pulses of jet lag. (I had left my friend Bernie Breitbart only hours ago. He had driven me from Princeton to the Newark Airport.) It was at this point that the tears came.

I excused myself and visited a friend in Santa Cruz until about 7:00. I wasn't up to being in Matsko's house while the deed was done and the body was carted away.

During the next several days, though old friends kept telling me I looked "wonderful," I didn't feel it. A sadness pervaded me in Aptos, in Santa Cruz, and at Stevenson College on the UCSC campus, where I had been elected an Honorary Fellow years ago, and where I now began writing in an office while living in Aptos. Passage of time, with its inevitable changes; in some cases, due to retirement; in others, to death. I involuntarily mourned for two men I had been close to: for a very witty and humorous professor who had died slowly of colon cancer; and for another, also very witty, and given to sly gallows humor, who had been taken rapidly by brain cancer.

However, this mood soon passed, and I socialized not only with California friends but with some from the East who either happened to be in California or who came to see me. Among the latter were Erik and Molly and Bernie, with whom I tried to share the area's great natural beauty, from Half Moon Bay in the north to Big Sur in the south. I also tried to show them how extraordinarily beautiful the UCSC campus is. Meanwhile I was regularly power-walking, and still slowly regaining strength and endurance that had been lost to radiotherapy.

SEPTEMBER 15, 1993, SANTA CRUZ, CALIFORNIA. I love Santa Cruz and the natural environs of this region. For example, I'm very familiar with Point Lobos just south of Carmel, which Edward Weston, a great American photogapher, used as the setting for a wonderful portfolio, *My Camera on Point Lobos*. I knew him when Joan and I lived in Carmel during the summer of 1954 and when I often and for long hours spent time on Lobos. He had Parkinson's then, and was hoping to have a book of his female nudes published. And I myself used Point Lobos as a literary setting for my novel *The Authentic Death of Hendry Jones*, which was made into the movie *One-Eyed Jacks*, starring Marlon Brando and produced and directed by him. I'm equally familiar with Año Nuevo, up the coast from Santa Cruz, where elephant seals breed.

There being no prostate cancer support group in town to my knowledge, I joined a general cancer support group in Newtown, California, whose meetings are held at St. Christina's Hospital every Wednesday afternoon. I've attended two, the second being today. There were about fifteen people present at each. Marcela, the temporary facilitator, who has reddish-brown hair, is immense. She gives the impression of carrying an enormous belly on a tricycle beneath her tentlike dress; but her face, neck and arms aren't large in proportion to the rest of her. She's intelligent, empathetic, gentle, soft-spoken.

Wendy, with Hodgkin's disease, has a pretty moon face, and soft blue eyes. At my first meeting she wore no wig, revealing very short blonde hair. Today she had a long blonde one. Sheila has lung cancer that metastasized to her brain. She had a brain operation. She speaks intelligently and courageously about herself. She wears a reddish, long wig. Lloyd has liver and pancreatic cancer. His long dark hair and his heavy, full beard look virile. Despite his beard, I sense his cheeks are hollow and that he clenches his jaws. He avoids eye contact and speaks in monosyllabic grunts. How old is he? In his mid-forties? How long is he likely to live? His gray-haired wife, Bunny, who has a pleasant face, seems much more mature than he.

Hilda, in remission with lymphoma, like Wendy has a moon face. She has very short brown hair (new growth). She frequently laughs and giggles. She was scheduled to have an operation last Wednesday, but it was canceled because she's doing so well.

"I'm having trouble dealing with this good news," she said seriously.

She read aloud a letter from a female group member, who sent regards to specific persons, noting their troubles in great detail and astonishing the group by her memory. Hilda has a slightly foreign-sounding accent, something heavier than American. She read well in poor light, rarely stumbling. Jeff, her companion (huge body, small head), was all smiles in his pride of her.

A lean Aussie of about fifty described himself as a lung cancer survivor and told an anecdote in his Aussie twang. Planning a trip to Australia, he had had a MedicAlert type of medallion engraved, which warned he had only a left lung. He had gone home and shown it proudly to his wife, who reminded him his left lung had been surgically removed.

"I'm Sandra," said a handsome, gray-haired woman (slit of a mouth, strong white teeth). "I'm here on behalf of my husband, Luke. He has squamous cell carcinoma. They discovered it as a lump in his throat. It had already metastasized. They haven't given him much longer to live. As a last-ditch effort they attached a pump to his arm, with a tube. They put him on heavy chemotherapy; at home. About 3:00 A.M. the other night he gets out of bed, goes to the kitchen and cuts the tube with a kitchen knife. The pump falls to the floor. He returns to the bedroom and rips the tube out of his arm. I awake, see the blood, and think I'm in a nightmare."

She cried softly. I liked her looks, facial language, courage. I felt stirrings of something like love for her.

"I take him to the ER," she continued after drying her eyes with a tissue. "A new tube and pump are attached. Then Poison Control tells me I can't go home for at least a day and a half, because the pump has poisoned the house. What am I to do? Go to a motel in the middle of the night? How can I cope there? I took him home."

"What emotional and psychological pain these people have endured and are enduring," I thought. "I'm an innocent by comparison."

Aside from myself, a man named Henry Trout is the only one in the group with prostate cancer. In mid-May (four months earlier), at forty-eight (relatively young for this cancer), he was diagnosed in both lobes. Stage: B2. PSA: 7. Gleason grade: 2+3. He's of middle height, handsome, married, and looks in good shape physically. Dr. Morgan, his Newtown oncologist, urged him to have an immediate prostatectomy; and, according to Trout, offered him the option of going on Lupron and Eulexin for six months "to shrink the tumor." Dr. Morgan didn't recommend radiation, because, as he explained, Trout is too young for it; there isn't a long enough survival time.

Instead of following Dr. Morgan's advice, Trout has been waiting, hoping to cure his cancer with herbal therapy and weight loss (the latter "to help starve the tumor"; he said he needs to lose thirty-five pounds). He's also considering having cryosurgery at the University of California at San Diego, where, he said, "the cost is very reasonable." He likes the idea of cryosurgery because it's less invasive than a prostatectomy, with less danger of impotence and incontinence. He's especially worried about the possibility of becoming impotent.

"You've waited four months since diagnosis," I said to him today. "If the cancer leaves the gland, you'll run out of options. You won't be able to have either surgery or radiation. You'll have to have hormone therapy, which will make you impotent."

"Not if I take it for only six months," he responded.

His overweight wife, Diana, said bitterly, "We haven't waited. We've been going the herbal route. Morgan refuses to give Henry a prescription for a PSA to see if the herbs have worked. We're pissed at Morgan. He's interested in only one thing—making money."

I wanted to say, "Wake up, man, before it's too late! You're concerned about impotence, but impotence may be the least of your problems if you run out of options through dillydallying."

Finally, I said to him this afternoon when I was briefly alone with him, "If I were you, I'd have an immediate prostatectomy." He seemed to take the statement casually, smiling gently as usual.

SEPTEMBER 22, 1993, SANTA CRUZ. Cancer support group meeting in Newtown. Running into Hilda (lymphoma) in the parking lot, I accompanied her to the conference room on the second floor of the brown wooden building, she informing me she had just visited Wendy (Hodgkin's disease) in the hospital because Wendy's white blood count had dropped too low. Several people, including Marcela, the temporary facilitator, were already present.

Bunny, Lloyd's spouse (Lloyd was the man with liver and pancreatic cancer), began the meeting by announcing, "Lloyd's at home. He's all right." Gray-haired, slender, wearing an old blue blouse, old blue jeans and scuffed athletic shoes, she said, "The woman who's his chief supplier of pot was busted today by the sheriff's office. She grew just half a dozen plants in her back yard, mostly to help people like Lloyd, suffering from intense pain. One officer said to her, 'I guess you'll have to *buy* the stuff this year.' I'm furious! I hope *I'll* get busted, so I can have my angry puss on national TV. Pot has been keeping Lloyd alive. At

175

one point the doctors gave him two weeks to live. He couldn't hold anything down because of pain. The drugs just didn't do it for him. With pot his pain disappeared, he started eating, he put on weight! We can't afford to go out and buy high-quality stuff. Lloyd's supplier also supplied the pot to make brownies for Luke, Sandra's husband."

"Is homegrown pot as good as the stuff you can buy?" somebody asked.

"Better," said Bunny, speaking intensely, and staring. "I'm putting out a call for anybody who can suggest a new and inexpensive source of the stuff."

Someone assured her *she* had ways and means. Other members murmured similar sentiments. Bunny announced that through the kindness of friends, she and Lloyd would soon make a week's trip back home to Oklahoma City. "I'm sorry I have to leave so soon. I need to take care of him," she added, and left.

Henry Trout entered the large conference room with a vague, distant smile, as if in response to a very private joke, and walked to a chair with a seemingly new, rambling, dancing, curving, rocking body language. His thick gray hair had been cut so short it now resembled a short-haired dog's. Was this the Henry Trout I knew? And where was his angry wife? Hilda's friend, Jeff, leaned back in his chair, tilting it onto its back legs and looking down his nose through his glasses; easier that way to support his great belly. He patted Hilda's thigh. Marcela asked us to identify ourselves.

When her turn came (next to last), the woman on my immediate right, a newcomer, stout, probably in her late fifties, with a tight mouth, said, "I'm Fay. I had a mastectomy last October, and some of the lymph nodes were removed. I don't think the cancer spread. I've always had weak disks in my neck and back. I had a pulmonary embolism because of bed rest due to the mastectomy. It required still more bed rest. So my posture muscles, which I had tried hard to keep strong to protect my disks, became very weak. I'm sure I'll need to have a disk fused in my neck. The pain will be terrible. It's almost worse than the cancer. I'm in pain a lot of the time. Frankly, I'm frightened. And I'm *very* low in funds. I have two boys. One of them and his wife are living with me for a while. I've always been the giver in my family. I've rarely asked for help. I never thought *I'd* need help. And now I need help. I need help. And I don't know where to turn. And I feel guilty, because my cancer is nothing compared to yours."

Fay wept. Tempted to cry myself, I patted her upper back. She seemed not to notice. "Does anyone have a tissue?" she asked in embarrassment. A tissue was relayed around the room to her.

"We've *been* there," said Sheila to her. Sheila was the lady whose lung cancer had gone to her brain. "We know what it's like. Last night I felt just like you're feeling now. Last week when I saw my doctor he palpated my back, and at one point pressed hard. That night I felt pain in one of my ribs, and I've felt it ever since. I'm afraid it's the cancer again. I hope it's a broken rib, because the pain came suddenly. I thought I was doing well, and now there's this new thing to worry about."

"They told me I didn't need an operation, because I was doing so well," said Hilda to Fay, smiling. "That was less than two weeks ago. And now they're not sure. It's hard to be sure of anything anymore."

"Can somebody tell something funny?" asked Marcela. "We need laughter."

"Well," said Henry Trout, "I went to a lab and asked for my autopsy report instead of my biopsy report." He made a face indicating chagrin.

"Sheila," Marcela said, "tell your PSA story."

Sheila laughed. "Once," she said, "while meeting with Dr. Adler, I said, 'I have a feeling you're keeping something important from me.' He looked surprised. 'What am I keeping from you?' he asked. I said, 'What are my PSAs?' He laughed and explained. I hadn't realized PSAs are special to the prostate."

"I'm sorry I took up so much of your time," said Fay when the laughter subsides.

Marcela turned to the man on Fay's right, whom I hadn't seen before, and nodded, indicating it was his turn to speak. He was tall, slender, with a pale face that suggested old ivory. The cast of his forehead and nose reminded me of Thomas Mann, the German novelist: vertical brow, nose thrust out as if to slice the wind.

"I'm Maury," he said in a deep voice. "I haven't been here in some time, because I didn't feel I was getting enough out of a support group. I have pancreatic cancer. It was diagnosed last Christmas. It had spread. I was given only a short time to live. I've had chemotherapy, radiation and surgery."

His leanness, voice and measured cadences reminded me of a friend who died of leukemia in his seventies.

"I'm getting by now by eating sensibly," continued Maury. "I don't eat much. But what I eat is wholesome. I don't smoke or drink. I've lost a lot of weight, but my weight seems to have stabilized. I'm no longer seeing doctors. I don't find such intervention useful any longer. I'm no longer interested in finding out where I stand. Except for painkillers, I no longer take medication of any kind. I let my body tell me what it needs. I'm content to live from day to day and week to week."

He was a grave presence, not only because of his illness but because of his slow, resonant speech. I was impressed by how courageous and graceful these people were.

Jill, probably in her early sixties, who always looked very sober and who wore a blonde, roundish, curly, wig-looking wig, said, "A male friend suddenly said to me the other day, 'That's an interesting topknot you have.' He wouldn't have said that to a man. It made me bitter for a couple of days."

Sympathizing with her, Brigid and Sheila exposed their stubbled heads, Brigid by removing her little white turban, Sheila by taking off her long, reddish, natural-looking wig.

"There's a tradeoff," said Brigid, laughing. "My hair's no longer gray."

"And mine's coming out straight," Sheila said. "It was curly before."

Wigless Hilda, whose hair suggested a fashionable "boy's" look, said, "My hair is different now both in color and texture." Gently touching her scalp with two fingers, she added, "I have a small male-pattern bald spot on my crown now."

Sheila noted two male-pattern bays that had appeared since her hair's return.

"I'd remove my wig too, except it's pinned onto my hair that's coming back," explained Fay.

"I never would have guessed you're wearing a wig," said Sheila admiringly. Her comment was echoed by Brigid and Hilda.

"Good! That makes me feel a lot better!" cried Fay.

"I've been very concerned about the passage of time," said Brigid suddenly to Henry Trout. "It seems to me you're waiting much too long to make a decision."

At Marcela's request, Henry explained his situation for Fay and Maury.

"Why do you want to hang on to your prostate?" asked Maury. His blunt, almost brutal tone surprised me.

"I don't want to hang on to it," Henry replied in his soft, gentle tone, smiling. "I'm considering cryosurgery. Most of the gland will probably be destroyed by that."

"Cryosurgery?"

Apparently Maury had never heard of it. Henry haltingly, nervously explained, with side glances, vague smiles, twitching of feet, intertwining and disengaging of hands.

"Why don't you stop researching? Why don't you do surgery?" asked Maury.

"I don't want to panic. Anyhow, my doctor told me my tumor is slow-growing."

Convinced I mustn't keep silent on the issue, that I must try to budge Henry from the dangerous game he had been playing for four months, I addressed the group in general and Brigid in particular, glancing at Henry from time to time.

"Henry told me his Gleason number. It's 5 on a scale of 2 to 10," I said. "It does not indicate a timid, slow-growing tumor. If it were a 2 or a 3, he might watchfully wait. But even then, given his relatively young age in terms of prostate cancer, and his probably still strong production of testosterone, I doubt he should go on waiting. Watchful waiting may be a strategy best suited to men in their late sixties or early seventies."

The group was silent, attentive. Henry didn't seem offended by my candor. After the meeting, chatting with him outside, I gathered he was into herbal medicine and therapy.

"Did your father and/or your brother have prostate cancer?" I asked.

"No."

"Why did Dr. Morgan prescribe Lupron? Why not do surgery at once?"

"Lupron will shrink the tumor, maybe even make surgery unnecessary."

Fay, the woman whose back I had patted, joined us and said to me, "Thanks for the physical support. It mattered a lot."

Marcela, the substitute facilitator, called me at home this evening to say, "I want to thank you for your contribution to the group." She said she and others of the group had spoken to Henry about his delay in reaching a decision, Sheila and Hilda having gone so far as to say, "We're fighting for our lives, while you're playing with yours." A cancer support group chiefly supports by pooling information, by sharing concern, and by letting members speak freely about themselves. Above all, such a group stresses survival.

Henry's house is on fire, yet he's still fiddling. What's the group's responsibility?

Eleven

September 29 to October 24, 1993

SEPTEMBER 29, 1993, SANTA CRUZ. Seventeen people were present at the cancer support group meeting in Newtown this afternoon, including Marcela, the substitute facilitator, and now Arthur, the regular one. I sometimes compared the two groups I belonged to. Conservative New Jersey (King City); and laid-back California (Newtown). Cancer limited to men; and general cancer, with women outnumbering men in the Newtown group.

Wendy was there! Sheila was there! Hilda was there! They weren't in the hospital! "Great to see you, Wendy!" said someone. "What was your white count?"

"Point 5," replied Wendy quietly. Her light brown hair looked crewcut. She wasn't wearing her wig.

"What's it now?"

"3.5, which isn't too bad."

"How do you feel?"

"Still very tired."

"And you, Hilda?" somebody else asked.

"I'm still in remission." Hilda's large male companion, smiling proudly, patted her shoulder.

"Sheila, how are *you*?" asked somebody.

"My rib *was* fractured," Sheila replied.

Loud clapping by the group. Cancer's paradox: a fractured rib as good news.

These strong feelings of concern between group members, at times amounting to worry, were authentic and realistic. Not surprisingly, real closeness had developed between these people who were sharing common hardships and tragedies. I myself had lost some sleep worrying about Henry Trout in particular. In addition to having a form of cancer in common with him, I liked him. I liked his soft manner; his body language; his friendliness.

And I was interested in his "cancer narrative," as it were, and experienced a kind of suspense regarding it. He was doing something that I considered very risky; and his physician held a similar view. What was going to happen to Henry? At what point, if ever, would he act on his case? Would his cancer go to bone, or would he somehow beat the odds? How long could he go on watchfully waiting, if that was what he was doing? He was forty-eight, a stripling where prostate cancer was concerned. If he were sixty-eight, it would be another matter.

Henry, sitting beside me, informed me that last week was Prostate Cancer Awareness Week, and that he had called in to a radio show, had spoken briefly with a Dr. Sheeran, and had seen Dr. Sheeran at St. Christina's Hospital for a free digital, and had had blood drawn for a free PSA. As usual, Henry spoke very softly, leaning forward.

"I told Sheeran I'm considering taking Lupron and Eulexin," he said. "Sheeran said, 'Who told you about Lupron and Eulexin?' I said, 'Dr. Morgan.' He said, 'Pay no attention to him. They have nothing to do with you. Have surgery *now*.' I'm going to see the VA first before making up my mind."

"What's your PSA, based on the free test?"

"It's not ready yet. It may take a while. I'll get another at the VA."

How long would Henry go on stalling? I imagined a man standing on the edge of a cliff, the earth crumbling under him, and yet I wasn't allowed to grab him. But he was an adult, with the right to be self-destructive.

Sandra wheeled her husband Luke in, terminally ill with metastasized squamous cell carcinoma. I hadn't seen him before. Glancing occasionally at him, I remembered the terrible scenes she had described—Luke, hallucinating in the kitchen at 3:00 A.M., using a kitchen knife to sever the tube connecting his vein to the chemotherapy pump; Luke in the bedroom, ripping the tube stump out of his arm; Sandra, waking up, seeing him, feeling she was in a nightmare; and the pump on the kitchen floor, pumping away, poisoning the house.

Seated in the wheelchair (faded, shoulder-length, gray-brown hair; faded killer mustache; high brown boots; one leg crossed), he looked small, curled up, gave the impression of being in a fetal position. We were all ghosts, but he was farther down the road. Mostly he was silent. When he spoke, his voice sounded as if it was coming from a little speaker. Was the tight white band around his throat related to his cancer? What had he been like as a four-year-old, full of gorgeousness, love, bounce? I thought of Annie, my granddaughter, four and a half, beautiful, and restless with twitchy muscles. Sandra, handsome, graying, smiling, said, "I'm so glad he was willing to come," and began to cry softly as she glanced first at him, then at the rest of the group. He whispered something comforting to her.

Arthur the facilitator told about his and his wife's recent trip to Germany, Austria and Switzerland. He had brought a couple of bars of Swiss chocolate to the meeting, which he now sent clockwise around the large conference room. The room was warm, the chocolate warmer, and there were no napkins, so people soon had gluey brown fingers. Maury (pancreatic cancer) slipped quietly into the room. And Patty, a newcomer, tall, lean, fit, now also joined us. She didn't seem like one of us. Had she strayed into the wrong room? She seemed too young, and too sexually attractive, to be here. She had too much long leg and too much luxuriant brown hair. What was her tiny, puckered mouth signaling? Or her staring blue eyes behind thick lenses?

Then she told her story: twenty-eight, she had recently discovered a lump in one of her breasts, and two weeks ago it had been found to be cancerous. She asked for advice now on how to set up her priorities. Group members, chiefly women, urged her to be accompanied by someone when she went to San Francisco for tests and results.

Brigid, removing her turban to show hair that was little more than a stubble, told what a blur she had been in when she had received *her* cancer news. "I went to my car. I hammered against the steering wheel. I cried. I was angry. Why me? I found myself driving down the highway. I had no idea how I got there. I told myself, 'You have no business driving by yourself like this.'"

Patty made notes with a pen. Marcela, the substitute facilitator, removed black slippers to cool stockingless feet. Fay (small face; large hams; a manner of speaking too forcefully for a relative newcomer) reported that she had gone to a hair stylist, gotten a boy's cut and had dispensed with her wig. The three wigged women commented admiringly about how much hair she had. Jill, the stolid lady with the round, blonde wig and the uterine cancer from which, presumably, she was in remission, said little.

"Have you ruled out surgery?" Arthur suddenly asked Henry Trout, tilting his thick gray head back and glancing down his nose through glasses.

Smiling shyly, Henry leaned forward to speak, revealing extra weight on his hips and back. "No. I'm still opening doors," he replied.

"Did you two discuss your cancer?" Arthur asked me.

"Yes. I told Henry what I think."

Arthur didn't pursue my remark's implications. As the meeting ended, Henry went over to Patty the newcomer and spoke with her. Maury and I left the building together. Maury wore gray sweats, and running shoes. "I've found that being curious about one's cancer is helpful in dealing with it," he remarked. "At the hospital I asked many questions. And went on grand rounds."

He smiled while saying this, and a pleasant light entered his speckled, light-brown eyes.

October 6, Santa Cruz. Fifteen people present at the support group meeting, including Arthur the facilitator. Marcela was absent.

"I was surprised by a call from a pharmacy, informing me to pick up my prescription," Henry immediately told me. "Dr. Morgan phoned it in. Lupron and some Eulexin pills. His nurse called and told me to come in tomorrow for my first Lupron shot. I bought the stuff. Morgan caught me by surprise."

At Arthur's request, people introduced themselves, going clockwise around the room. Sheila, the pale lady with the strong nose, intellectual face and long, reddish wig, was first. "I'm Sheila. I had a brain operation to remove a tumor. The doctors decided it had had to come from somewhere else, so they did exploratory surgery. They found a tumor in a lung. They removed it. They found one in a rib. They removed that too. I'm in remission."

Wendy was next. Her cheeks were round, as if from cortisone use, and always seemed to be blushing. Her expression, as usual, was bland. Her blue eyes stared. She was wigless. Her short blonde hair was thin. "I have Hodgkin's, which I think is in remission," she said. "Sometimes I'm so tired I can hardly pick up even my smallest child. This Friday will be my last chemotherapy session."

We all cried, "Congratulations!" and clapped.

Fay said, "I'm Fay. I had a mastectomy. And three crushed cervical disks. I'm afraid a fourth will soon need fusing. Both my parents were alcoholics. I was abused in various ways, including sexually, from the time I was born until I was thirteen. I was a mess. I hoped this time at group meeting I wouldn't cry. But here I am, crying. [She wiped her eyes and nose with a tissue.] The other day Dr. Harris said I'm addictive. I resent that. He doesn't know me well enough to call me that. I'm going to tell him so. I cried. I take a lot of Percocet, but it's for my disk pain. I'm in pain a lot of the time. I'm not addictive. He's so unfair."

"It's all right to cry, Fay," said Hilda. "We all cry sooner or later."

"I'd *tell* him," Lois said. Lois had short gray hair, a squarish face and seamed skin as if from too much smoking. She spoke in a flat, "tough" voice. "I'm Lois. I'm here on behalf of my husband, Jimmy. He doesn't have much longer to live. He's down to 128. His blood pressure is 60 over 40. He falls and hurts himself because it's so low. I'm not sure how much longer I can hang on. But I'll do my best."

Much attention was paid to Patty the newcomer, who, wearing shorts, sat with her heels on her chair seat, hugging her well-defined legs.

"How you doing?" Arthur asked her.

"I'm having a very bad time," she said quietly. Her mouth, born small, seemed smaller than it had last week. Her stare behind thick lenses was clouded.

"What's your situation?" he asked. A long pause. "It's time for me to make a decision," she said. "Should it be a lumpectomy? A mastectomy? I'm not sure if a lymph node is affected. Chemotherapy will shrink the tumor before the operation. But shrinking it may hide the node's real condition."

"Try a needle biopsy?" suggested Sheila. Patty, whose gaze seemed focused beyond the room, didn't reply.

"I'm Jill," said Jill quietly. "I was diagnosed with cervical cancer in February. I'm having chemotherapy. People kept thinking cervical cancer is in the neck, so now I call it uterine cancer."

Brigid, wearing her gay little turban, said with a smile, "I have ovarian cancer. I had *three* gynecologicals!" She gestured broadly to indicate hospital personnel suddenly lifting her hospital gown to examine her crotch. "I was so grateful for medical attention I'd have walked down the corridor naked if ordered to. I've had chemotherapy. I'm in remission."

As the session was about to end and people stood up, Hilda reminded the group that this was my last meeting with them, and she came over to me and handed me a small bouquet of mums and zinnias, together with a card with my first name written on it. Hugging me, she started to cry. I was surprised, embarrassed and bewildered. I had never had a bouquet handed me. Why was she hugging me so hard? Did she feel my going was like a death, and that death was too intimate a stalker here? Holding the flowers, I studied her eyes. We hugged again.

Sheila, strong-nosed, pale, shorter than I expected, also hugged me hard. Looking pained, her face broke into tears. We separated, then hugged again. Remembering her fractured rib, I was careful not to squeeze hard. I kissed the right side of her head, then realized I was kissing her long, reddish wig. My eyes were turning watery, my jaw was trembling. What was expected of me? What should I do? They didn't even know my last name. Brigid, lean, warm, hugged me and wept. Fay followed suit. I found myself crying softly.

After the meeting, Lois, who usually looked and sounded tough at meetings, surprised me by unburdening herself when we were alone together outdoors. I had just said good-bye to Henry Trout. Strongly shaking hands, we had emotionally told each other to take care.

"I need some life for myself!" Lois began suddenly. "I can't go out to socialize. People are reluctant to visit us. We postponed two trips last October. I'm cut off! A friend of mine said, 'Can't you *do* something?' Do *what*? I can't just throw Jimmy out the window. My pastor phoned and said, 'Call if you need me.' I said, 'What do you mean?' He said, 'Call if you have a problem.' I have 500 problems a *day*! I just wish Jimmy would get it over with! He's down to 128 from 215. Sometimes I think, 'Either get better or die!' I sound horrible but I'm near the end of my rope! I have absolutely no life of my own! Young Jimmy visited us recently. He had a hard time being parted from his dad. He kept clinging to him. His dad said, 'Go! Live your life! I know you love me. I love you too. We'll surely meet again.' Yet Laurie, our only daughter, hasn't seen her dad in months. She hasn't even called! I'll never, ever, forget what she's done to me and Jimmy. I don't know about other people's faith, but Jimmy and I are Christians, we go to church on Sunday and donate. Why does this happen to *us*? I can't take much more! I'll never, ever, forgive her!"

"How old is she?" I asked.

"Thirty-two."

"Has she ever been married?"

"No. And she's a nurse! She ought to know better!"

"When Jimmy is gone, I think the wound between you and Laurie will heal."

"Think so?" asked Lois, looking puzzled and hopeful.

I returned to Princeton on October 9. On the 11th, roughly four months after I completed radiation therapy, I had blood drawn at the King City hospital for a PSA and an acid phosphatase. Although I was optimistic, I was aware of possibly harboring some radiation-resistant cancer cells as well as some metastasis, so I braced myself against the chance of still having a high PSA. Three days later Dr. North surprised me by calling to say, "I have your new PSA, and I don't feel it's fair to hold back good news."

"Great! What is it?"

"6.2. Down from 16.4 before therapy, and 8.9 a month after therapy."

"Terrific!"

"I'm very pleased and excited. I'm always pleased when I see the PSA dropping after therapy. 6.2 may turn out to be your baseline. It depends on the gland's volume, which can be determined from the ultrasound. I'm referring to the PSA density: the PSA divided by the volume."

"Why is there a six-month lag between the end of radiation therapy and the onset of any radiation-caused impotence?" I asked. "Is it due to damage to the erectile nerves?" The questions had been on my mind recently.

"It's more likely to be due to a vascular phenomenon, though some direct damage to the nerves sometimes does occur. The capillaries feeding the nerves may be scarred or otherwise impaired, and this eventually damages the nerves. How are you in that department?"

"Fine."

"Excellent."

I was excited by my PSA news and by Dr. North's pleasure in it. The radiation had worked for the first four months! All that lying on the treatment bed under the mysterious linac; all those rays streaming mysteriously through me and bouncing madly off floor, ceiling, walls, door; all that wondering what the PSA would be. All had come to some good, at any rate so far. In the evening, aware that friends and relatives were worried about me, I enjoyed sharing my news. "Enjoy it while you can," I thought, "because in cancer, who knows truly where you're heading?"

I have an appointment with Dr. North next Monday, the 18th. What will he find during the digital? Has the tumor shrunk again?

OCTOBER 18, 1993. Dr. North, tall, dark-bearded, smiling, friendly, looking fit, wearing a white coat, remarked, "You look great!" when I met with him today.

"That's what people said in Santa Cruz who had heard about my cancer. They sounded surprised, as if they had expected to see a walking cadaver."

"I assumed you would do well, from the way you were handling the therapy."

"What's my acid phosphatase? I gather many doctors are skeptical about acid phosphatase these days. Daniel Redmont said he pays little attention to it."

"2.4. Down from 3.9."

"What do you foresee for my final post-therapy PSA?"

"My guess is . . . about 4.5."

"Can my right hip pain have been caused by the radiation?"

"When you get on in years and there's maybe a bit of arthritis, the radiation through your hip doesn't help."

After doing a digital he said, "If I didn't know your case, if my finger didn't remember what it had felt before, I'd conclude that the gland feels normal. The protuberance is gone. All I feel is a bit of scarring . . . maybe."

"What about the gland's size?"

"It's not especially large. When will you see Lew Gilroy?" [My urologist.]

"Around the end of November, when I'll return to my home in Princeton from a stay at the MacDowell Colony."

"What's that?"

"It's the oldest artists' colony in the country. It's located in Peterborough, New Hampshire. I'm going there for a month. When I get back I'll get another PSA, this one maybe on Dr. Gilroy's new machine."

"Keep in mind that PSA machines differ. If you get a PSA, for example, of 6.4 on Dr. Gilroy's machine (instead of the hospital's most recent 6.2), don't be upset."

I told him about the Newtown, California, general cancer support group and how candidly, gracefully and bravely they behaved, and I spoke about Henry Trout. When I mentioned Trout's relatively young and therefore dangerous age for prostate cancer (forty-eight), Dr. North drew his breath in sharply and frowned, but said nothing.

"When do I see you next?" I asked.

"Normally, in six months. But because we're friends and I enjoy seeing you, let's make it three. We never charge for follow-up visits, so there's no concern on that score."

OCTOBER 24, 1993, THE MACDOWELL COLONY, PETERBOROUGH, NEW HAMPSHIRE. The MacDowell office informs me this is my tenth stay here. I first came in the fall of 1951, and was last here in the spring of 1977, shortly after leaving Antarctica for the third time. Having recently published two separate, quality-paperback novellas, I came here a week ago to work on a third, *The Left Eye Cries First,* my hope being to produce a hard-cover book comprising all three. But as soon as I settled in after the long drive northward in a heavy rain, I realized I was too preoccupied with writing *Adam's Burden* to do both, so I shelved the idea of dealing with the novella, a decision that was approved by the Colony's resident director.

I haven't tried self-hypnosis yet in connection with my cancer, having been too busy with other matters, but I must do so, and this is an excellent place and time for it. My goals are:

(1) to kill any "normal" cancer cells in the prostate that may have eluded radiation;

(2) to kill any radiation-resistant cancer cells that may exist;

(3) to attack all secondary cancers that may have been caused by X-ray penumbras, as well as those possibly caused by X rays that ricocheted off the walls of the treatment room after penetrating me;

(4) to cleanse the urethra, seminal vesicles, nearby lymph nodes and all bones of any prostate cancer cells;

(5) to reduce the gland's size, as well as that of any remaining tumor or protuberance;

(6) and to avoid impotence.

I know from experience how to do self-hypnosis. To explain why I have faith in the process, I'll describe my sole and successful encounter with it.

In April 1980 I had a growth on the lower lid of my left eye which I considered having removed by my eye doctor, Dr. Sieswerda, whom I saw annually at the Eye Institute of the Columbia-Presbyterian Medical Center in New York. Calling it a tumor, Dr. Sieswerda said surgery would require hospitalization for two days, and he urged me not to have a dermatologist do it in an office, for the result could be ugly. Joan, after watching a New York medical hypnotherapist on TV, suggested I see him, so I met with Herbert Krieger, M.D., on April 10 and decided to try to remove the growth by self-hypnosis, a more conservative approach. Dr. Krieger gave me some tests, pronounced me talented as a hypnosis subject, and taught me how to do the necessary self-hypnosis. I agreed to report to him in four weeks.

My ground-floor study was (and is) surrounded on three sides by a yard containing ivy, a lawn, and cedars and maples. Though the exposure is northern, light could still distract me, so I darkened the study before each self-hypnosis session. I always sat in the same chair, arms outstretched on the chair arms, my feet resting on a canvas camp stool. Closing my eyes and rolling them upwards a bit, I took a deep breath and exhaled slowly, counting from 1 to 5 while imagining helium entering my left arm as if the arm were a balloon. That was how I always began.

My arm rose on its elbow and stayed like that during the session. My wrist was limp. My breathing changed dramatically, becoming deep, steady and very pleasant. During self-hypnosis I was often keenly aware of my pulse. At times I fell asleep, but even if I didn't, when I ended the session I felt refreshed, as though by a profound nap. I quit the session by slowly lowering my arm while counting 3, 2, 1; resting my arm on the chair arm on 1; and opening my eyes.

At Dr. Krieger's suggestion I visualized a laser beam attacking the eyelid growth. I usually preferred an orange laser because it reminded me of molten iron. At times I imagined the growth heating up and smoking. A single color bored or distracted me, so I changed colors, switching to green or purple or yellow. The lasers seemed to stem from my head. Now and then I imagined speaking to them. "Attack the growth! Starve it! Burn it! Explode it! Make the flesh clean!"

On occasion I used a bundle of lasers. The attacking end had sharp points. Sometimes I attacked the eye as a whole, but this usually produced an unpleasant feeling in the eyeball. The attack wasn't continuous; it proceeded in pulses. I noticed that the laser pulsed in synch with my pulse. Before I started self-hypnosis the growth would sometimes itch and I would scratch it. During self-hypnosis it itched much more.

I called Dr. Krieger on May 12. "I wish I had taken photos as a benchmark at the beginning," I said. "It would make the process easier if I were sure I'm not deluding myself. Sometimes I can't be sure if I'm seeing progress. But on the whole I think I am."

"That's very encouraging," he said.

"After each session I feel so much better in general, very refreshed. And my memory and my mind feel sharper."

"That's what's called a spinoff. So you see, without knowing about it, it happened to you."

I told him about some right-eye discomfort I had recently had, and some floaters in that eye (bits of benign pigment associated with aging), and suggested a possible connection with rolling my eyes upwards at the start of each self-hypnosis session.

After listening carefully he said, "In my opinion there's no connection. In 20,000 cases there hasn't been one such episode related to the self-hypnosis. The rolling of the eyes is external to the vitreous. It involves only external muscles. By the way, it's not too late to take photos now."

"I'll take them."

"Report to me in four weeks. I'd like to follow your case. Your observations may be contributive. There's so very little known about the effects of mind on tissue."

I always sharply visualized the growth, usually looking down at it, and I saw the stabbing laser beams. One day I was positive I was seeing progress. Next day I was less certain. The third day I was sure I saw none. Were the presumed changes due to self-witchery? I began to suspect it was counterproductive to watch the tissue closely. I might become disappointed and thus weaken my faith in the process and thereby lose ground.

In my imagination the laser beam was not an abstraction. I saw its line, its color, and could observe it jiggle in the strange way a real laser does. At times, when I was tired, my mind wandered or I nodded. Changing laser color helped make a fresh start. I didn't try a white laser. White seemed too antiseptic, decent, kind. I didn't want a "nice" laser, I needed a "killer." One mid-May afternoon I used a blue laser for the first time. It was such a deep, beautiful blue.

For a while I saw two or three small black spots in the part of the growth I thought had shrunk a bit. These could have been dried blood resulting from tiny tears caused by my rubbing the eye when it itched. I believed, however, that they were due to a shrinking process, like that occurring in a shriveling apple. Noticing that boredom was a growing problem and that the laser colors were becoming vaguer, I tried a white laser for the first time to freshen things up. To my surprise, it worked. Sometimes I surrounded the white one with a bundle of fiery reds.

Toward the end of May I had much trouble focusing my eyes when I was at my desk or when I was reading. I thought this was due to the floaters in my right eye. (My right eye still troubled me after an attack of floaters that had occurred the previous fall as a result of vigorous garden work. There had never been any pain, but there was much distraction if a semi-opaque bit of matter floated in front of my retina. Dr. Sieswerda had said it might take a year or two for the eye to recover completely.) I phoned him now. He suggested cold compresses and said the floaters might have something to do with the problem, but that it probably had to do with simple blood-vessel aging.

Joan took two photos of the growth the morning of June 1, 1980. That day I had much trouble focusing. The following morning my left eye, the one without floaters, gave me a good deal of anxiety. There was some graininess in the image produced by the eye. And there was an obstruction in the pupil, which made it hard for me to see clearly. Also, the eye was unable to resolve a straight line. Instead, it broke the line down into a stream of tiny points that resembled a laser beam. And the area of difficult vision contained a new, yellowish pigment.

The situation hadn't occurred suddenly. Several times during self-hypnosis, when I was zapping the left eyelid with lasers, the center of the eye had gone into a brief spasm. Later, while I was in my bathroom, the walls of which were white, I had more than once seen a chain of blood vessels, as if they were projected by my left eye onto the wall. The morning of June 3, whenever I blinked my left eye I saw an image of a little ragged circle, tinted yellow, smack in the middle of the eyeball. Remembering that I had recently seen an hour-long TV program on lasers, it seemed to me more than coincidental that the simple, straight lines (the horizontal ones) of my calendar book should now resemble laser beams, should have that odd, airy, broken look of real lasers. The vertical lines, when observed by my left eye (the right one being shut), were fuzzy and not straight; they curved.

Could self-hypnosis have harmful effects? And if so, was this new condition of my left eye caused by my zapping it with imagined lasers? Almost nothing was specifically known about the mechanism of hypnosis, either the psychic part or the somatic one, and yet there was a widespread belief that hypnosis could only be beneficial, that there was some built-in system in us that kept it from doing us harm. On the other hand, there was simultaneously a growing sense that emotional depression could affect one's immune system and lower one's resistance even to cancer. It seemed to me such depression might be, in some respects, a form of self-hypnosis.

It was well known that hypnosis could raise blisters on healthy tissue. Could it also injure eye tissue? I was a gifted subject, according to Dr. Krieger. I had a well-developed visual imagination. And I was intense emotionally and perceptually. Did tiny eye muscles and capillaries grow tense when my mind told them their region was being zapped by lasers? It was true that lasers were being used for optic healing. Welding detached retinas into place was a well-known example. But I was sending lasers not to heal but to destroy, and although I usually directed them at the eyelid growth, often I sent them to the eye in general. With much tension resulting, had small hemorrhages occurred, or some distortion of the lens? I recalled now that I had never felt comfortable with the imagined beams going directly to my eyeball. When I considered all this I became certain the TV program, which showed many lasers, had stimulated me to zapping more vigorously than ever. After that program I would, when doing self-hypnosis, first see the ruby crystal, then the brilliant color, and then I'd send the gorgeous ruby beam.

The chief theme of my thoughts now was a cautionary one. Dr. Krieger didn't know how intense I could be; how strongly I could imagine visually; and how single-mindedly I could approach a project. I wondered if it wouldn't have been safer to direct me to use a less destructive force than a laser, or at any rate to advise me to be cautious in its use. Ah, but the idea of caution seemed counterproductive. Hypnosis works largely on faith. (Much of it seems to work because of a genetic predisposition, whatever that may mean.) In short, I thought, it may well be that hypnosis is a two-way street.

Once I had this idea firmly in mind, I resolved to reverse the destructive process I had subjected my left eye to. I stopped zapping the eye or its lid with lasers, and I undertook self-hypnosis sessions in which I told *both* closed eyes that they were cool, beautifully round, crystal clear, and that they saw exceedingly well. I started these sessions around noon of June 2. Also, I took to drinking large amounts of water to detoxify myself if that was needed, and to calm myself. (I had been unusually tense the past several days.)

By evening I thought I could see some progress. By late night I was convinced I could see more. The yellow pigment had disappeared. The ragged circle had closed up and become a whitish dot of decreasing size. The horizontal lines of my calendar (as I viewed them), although not entirely unbroken, were losing some of their airy laser quality. And the vertical lines were beginning to look straight. Next morning I could see more progress still. When I blinked my left eye I no longer saw even the large whitish dot. Nevertheless I phoned Dr. Sieswerda, who said I should see him. He was unaware of my self-hypnosis project.

He was a remote, very lean, very gentle man with a gentle smile, a poker back and slow, deliberate body movements. His cheeks were roundish, his voice slightly husky, his manner formal, efficient, methodical, unhurried. He gave me the impression of inhabiting another world. I had inherited him from an eye doctor who had retired. When I detailed my symptoms, he ascribed them to the normal process of aging; that is, to changes in the optic blood vessels. I wondered if this opinion was correct. Wasn't it odd, I asked myself, that I had never had such troubles with my eyes prior to self-hypnosis? He dilated my pupils and examined the back of both eyes. He said there was nothing wrong with them; the floaters in the right eye and some tiny ones in my left were normal for my age. My vision was fine, I didn't need a new prescription for glasses. I was greatly relieved.

Then I told him about my self-hypnosis sessions and my suspicion that self-hypnosis (or any kind of hypnosis, for that matter) was a double-edged sword, and that I might have injured my left eye by zapping it with imagined lasers.

"I agree," he said firmly, to my surprise. "There is no known medication that doesn't have some disadvantages. Hypnosis is a form of medication. It can be very beneficial in some instances, but it should be used with care."

I told him about the spasms in my left eye; the projected chain image on the bathroom wall; the ragged little circle with a yellowish pigment; the printed straight lines that to the left eye looked like laser beams. He took all of this seriously and urged me to proceed with caution in the use of self-hypnosis.

"You're lucky you didn't injure the retina," he said. "If you pay less attention to your eyes, it will help them to recover."

On June 9 I called Dr. Krieger as scheduled and reported that after eight weeks of self-hypnosis I still wasn't sure if I was making progress. I reminded him of the uncertainty of the growth's being wart tissue. "Shall I continue?" I asked.

"Yes. Persist. Sometimes it can take four or five months to see real improvement."

"My wife, Joan, yesterday, when photographing the eyelid, said the growth looks smaller. We've been taking photos at weekly intervals, and eventually, when they're developed, we'll be able to note improvement if there's any."

I didn't mention to him at this time my (and Dr. Sieswerda's) suspicion that I might have injured my left eye. I did ask him if it was possible to do harm with self-hypnosis.

"Hypnosis *can* do some harm if it's used mischievously, but it's unlikely," he responded. "And it's impossible in the way we're using it. I wish it could. There are a lot of people I'd like to injure."

We laughed.

I didn't do self-hypnosis for the next three or four weeks. In mid-July 1980, while on an extended visit to Santa Cruz, I happened to glance into a mirror and was startled to see how much smaller the eyelid growth had become since I had last studied it in Princeton. Skin creases under the lid that had been hidden for years were now clearly visible; and eyelashes that had been obscured or embraced by the growth were now, at last, free of it. The self-hypnosis had succeeded despite the lapse in my attention. When I studied the left eyelid with a magnifying glass in mid-October, I discovered that all traces of the lesion were gone.

No danger of surgical complications. No discomfort during the recovery process. No bandages. No bills for surgery, anesthesia, hospitalization. And not the slightest trace of a scar. The mysterious mechanism, directed by the brain, was able to work on a cellular level, and to distinguish the growth tissue from the normal tissue, and to kill it, and to cart it away internally like an expert garbage collector.

The reader will now perhaps better understand why, having had this experience with self-hypnosis, I was ready to try self-hypnosis for my cancer. After I finished writing the present narrative, a friend, reading it, asked me why I didn't try it earlier. The answer is: I don't know.

Twelve

October 25 to November 26, 1993

OCTOBER 25, 1993, MACDOWELL COLONY. The weather continues mild and beautiful. A soft, seducing afternoon now. Hard to stay indoors, but work must be done. There are twenty-three artists in residence here currently. They comprise poets, writers, composers, painters, a sculptor, a photographer and a presentation artist. Nothing to do here but work, and I'm perhaps doing too much of it. I haven't gotten close to anyone here yet. I wonder if age does it. This place is wonderful, and I have great quarters, but at my age one does get lonely. Also, I'm intent on pushing along with *Adam's Burden*.

OCTOBER 27. It's morning of a dark, rainy day. Last evening at dinner I sensed a general malaise, probably caused by the weather's quickly changing from beautiful and dry to cold and wet. Even young people complained they weren't feeling well. Three said it was chiefly due to too much partying and not enough sleep.

After dinner I played a couple of games of cowboy pool, a traditional game here, on the old, large, gracious table, with its fresh felt and decent, if old, cue sticks. It's a combination of pocket pool and billiards. The rules can seem complex, and I had forgotten some of them and had to have my memory refreshed by an elderly female composer who had watched me play in the old days and who, astonishingly, remembered them in every detail. "He's an expert!" she remarked dogmatically about me to a number of artists standing around to observe in the pool-table lights under the high rafters of the spacious wooden hall.

I hadn't held a cue stick in some eighteen years, and my eyes had suffered a sea change; as had my hands; and feet; and knees; and back. I expected my playing now would be disastrous, so was surprised to feel and see the skill returning well enough to sustain my dignity with a fairly proficient, young and ambitious male opponent, who, after being twice defeated, remarked affectionately, "The old guard refuses to stand aside!"

Walking with a flashlight over a sandy road back to my quarters after the games, I was suffused with old memories of the Colony, and with old "ghosts," people I had known well there, some now scattered across the nation, and some now dead.

I've just listened to Mozart's clarinet concerto (KV622) on my CD player to elicit a quiet mood after the loud breakfast conversation.

I begin self-hypnosis by sitting comfortably on a corner of the sofa, feet on a captain's chair, right arm on the sofa's arm, left arm on two pillows. But then I remove my bifocals and wristwatch because they may distract me. I close my eyes, roll them upwards a bit, take a deep breath and slowly exhale, counting to five while lifting my left arm on its elbow and imagining it's filling with helium. My first goal of the day is to reduce my prostate's size. By imagined compression? No, for though this would reduce volume, it wouldn't reduce weight, and the added density might exert pressure on the urethra and bladder. By using a roto-rooter? Seeing the roto-rooter turning in my mind's eye, I decide it's too primitive for delicate tissue. I'll do a TURP (transurethral resection of the prostate), but instead of using a mechanical device such as urologists use, I'll try a laser spinning on its longitudinal axis. A laser is more precise, accurate.

And so I imagine a beam of indifferent color entering my penis, urethra and prostate. At first the procedure feels uncomfortable. Cautious (my knowledge of human anatomy in this area is a mass of ignorance), I prefer this approach to penetrating my abdomen, for I'm unsure what organs, tissues and blood vessels may be affected by an external laser, and I dislike the idea of making an incision for a fiber-optic device.

What laser color shall I use? I try ruby; it's vivid. I quickly dislike it, for I imagine the gland's inside to be the color of blood, and I'd like to avoid confusing my inner vision with a ruby beam against a bloody background. I try white. But I've never actually seen a white laser, and this undercuts the imagined white laser's authority. Also, white feels too contrasty and invasive for the red gland. Trying an electric blue that reminds me of certain crevices in Antarctic ice, I'm satisfied. The blue laser spins on its longitudinal axis, microscopically vaporizing tissue. It spins slowly at first until I get my bearings. I must be careful not to remove too much tissue. I'm reminded of the way huge tunnels are built: the one between England and France; and the unfinished circular tunnel beneath Texas, meant for the now defunct superconducting supercollider.

My eyebrow itches. I ignore it. My chin itches. The itching grows more intense, as if to spite me. I mustn't suddenly open my eyes and drop my arm to scratch. It's important to respect the self-hypnosis process if I wish the process to respect me. So I leave it by the rules. Slowly counting 3, 2, 1, I lower my left arm. At 1 it rests on the pillows as I open my eyes. I scratch, then formally reenter the session. Soon the tip of my penis says, "I'm not sure I like this [the spinning laser]. It's too hot. It makes me squirm." So I use an imaginary analgesic salve to quiet it, and I continue treating the gland.

Can an imaginary laser, over time, harm such delicate tissue? I decide not to have a spinning laser inside my penis and urethra. I invent a special laser: only the part of it inside my gland spins. Soon I improve on this. (Why follow a standard TURP procedure? Isn't my self-hypnosis a physiological magic wand?) The laser's *source* is now inside the gland, so penis and urethra are spared the laser field.

Though I understand that the gland is complex, consisting of five histologically distinct lobes (two lateral; and anterior, posterior and median), I treat its inside as a simple tunnel, being reassured by my sense it has its own self-defensive mechanisms, overseen by the brain. Also, there are possibly some the brain has no control over or even knowledge of. In self-hypnosis I'm addressing levels older and more "profound" than either the brain or specific organ tissues; levels analogous to those that regenerate lost limbs in certain species, for example the salamander. In addition, my brain is the mediator between intention and prostatic tissues (but only partially; I sense means of communicating with the tissues directly), and will try to keep me from harming myself.

How does the vaporized material emerge from the gland? I sense it's part of my job, if I'm to succeed, to leave no question unanswered, once it has arisen, so I invent a fine suction tube that removes the material via the urethra and penis. At times, without my wishing it, hydraulic pressure seems to be exerted on all sides of the gland to speed the process of diminishing the gland's size. I stop it. Safer to keep the procedure simple. The blue laser, spinning at about four times a second, is more likely to succeed if left alone. It doesn't need help, especially from an unknown source. Its present rate of spin is comfortable. If the spinning speeds up I get too excited, distracted. If it slows down I begin to nod.

I experiment: can I do self-hypnosis while listening to Mozart's Piano Concerto No. 25? No; the music is too powerful; it disrupts visualization.

The session lasts about twenty minutes, as most of my sessions do. I do two or three a day, and on rare occasions four.

4 P.M. Another session. I visualize the prostate's location above and near my pubic bone; then the gland's cavity; then the rotating blue beam. Now the beam turns at about twice, not four times, a second; a comfortable rate. Is this because I'm not as energetic as I was in the morning? Doubling its speed, I make myself unhappy. I decide to let it do what it wants. I no longer use a suction tube. Merely imagining something entering my penis is unpleasant. And my past experience with self-hypnosis convinced me the body has its own system of garbage disposal. In any event, I'm only suggesting that the *size* of the inner cavity be decreased. The body's interpreters will transform my message into body language on a cellular scale. Some special control room will hopefully take care that only cells involved in age-related benign prostatic hypertrophy will be removed, by what mysterious process I leave it to the body in its wisdom to determine.

As I understand it, laser beams are linear, a fact I overlooked when I instructed a blue laser to spin on its longitudinal axis. So what I'm now doing is visualizing a sphere of blue laser beams rotating inside my prostate at a rate varying from twice to four times a second and gently, gradually, vaporizing tissue.

I've read that eunuchs don't get prostate cancer. They lack testicles to produce testosterone. What about the androgen (male hormone) produced by their adrenals? I've also read that some women, at high risk for breast cancer, have had their breasts removed as a preventive measure. Should men at high risk for prostate cancer have a prostatectomy?

OCTOBER 28, 1993, MACDOWELL COLONY. A lovely day, with clouds, but very windy. It's warmer in town, more sheltered. My spacious studio is full of light this morning. There's sunlight beyond my white curtains and the lacy tree masses. Other windows, almost floor to ceiling, are uncurtained. No sounds of traffic or planes. A door slams distantly, but only rarely, somewhere in the building. My small refrigerator buzzes unobtrusively except when it shudders loudly to a stop. The day is windy. Cold air seeps around the storm windows. Occasionally the heat goes on with a roar.

I intend to destroy all radiation-resistant cancer cells, assuming there were some to begin with. What color laser to use for a search-and-destroy mission, and how to highlight such cells? Inject the prostate with a chemical? Injection feels obnoxious. Equip the laser with a device that spots recalcitrant cells? Too complicated. I invent an ultraviolet laser (invisible to humans; ultraviolet because its wavelength is shorter and more intense than that of visible light) that can detect and vaporize such cells. The beam rummages among the prostatic lobes. A thought: what if, after all the radiation I've had, radiation-resistant cells are beginning to flourish? Will I need an orchiectomy? Hormone therapy? The laser darts energetically here and there. A cell suddenly vaporizes. Was it a recalcitrant one? A normal cancer cell damaged by X rays? A normal cancer cell overlooked by radiation? A benign cell?

Impotence as a possible radiation side effect; usually beginning about six months to two years after therapy. Do X rays, in addition to harming the erectile nerves and/or the capillaries supplying them with blood, also damage blood vessels directly involved in erection? Dr. North said being sexually active helps prevent (or delay?) impotence. "Use it or lose it," he advised. Is there a difference, in this respect, between heterosexual and homosexual activity? What about men without lovers? Does masturbation help prevent impotence? If so, does it help as much as intercourse? Is orgasm required, or is erection enough? Is all sexual activity beneficial to blood vessels that nourish the erectile nerves?

How to proceed with self-hypnosis to prevent radiation-caused impotence? But first, how to distinguish between this kind and the kind caused by aging? I assume that in age-caused impotence there is general deterioration of the erection mechanism, whereas in radiation-caused impotence only the erectile nerves are involved, so I decide to concentrate on the nerves. I don't know how many there are (I seem to recall there are two, one on each side of the prostate gland, each enclosed in a sheath), but they have to be within the standard radiation field, and also probably within the conedown field. I'll get at them through my lower abdomen, using a ruby laser harmless to skin.

In self-hypnosis for my eye I had an external target by which I could measure progress. I have no such help now. I'll never know to what extent self-hypnosis helps clear my prostate of cancer cells or helps prevent permanent damage to my erectile nerves. I'll have to go on faith alone.

I change my mind about the ruby laser. Instead, I imagine four long acupuncture needles, fresh from their packages, which I know from actual experience cause no pain. I insert them just above my pubic bone, two for each nerve, at the nerve's head and foot. The needles are skin deep; they're not meant to touch the nerves. Eyes shut, observing them, breathing deeply, I imagine them warming the area, increasing blood flow to it. My left arm tires from standing on its elbow. I briefly end the session to let it rest. I find myself nodding. I stop hypnosis until I'm nod-free.

Now I use a ruby laser to look for and attack stray "normal" cancer cells (as distinguished from radiation-resistant ones) and to destroy any remnant of a tumor-protuberance in my left prostatic lobe. What's the tumor's size? Dr. North thinks it's now only a bit of scar tissue, hard to detect digitally. I order the laser to remove scar tissue as well as any remaining cancer tissue. (I may as well be a big spender in this fantasy world.) The ruby laser is vivid in my mind's eye. I'm reminded of ruby lasers in the Oncology Center's simulation and treatment rooms. Remembering an actual laser helps me visualize one. I see its beam scurrying as it flushes out stray cells.

OCTOBER 29, MACDOWELL COLONY. Last evening I declined a party in the library beginning at 10:30, and went home and listened to Milladoiro (Galician Spanish folk music) on CD. This morning, refreshed, I'm happy to be concentrating on self-hypnosis. My only bone scan was done on March 4. My therapy began April 12. It was possible for prostate cancer cells to travel to bone (for which, I have read, such cells have a preference) between March 4 and the time when radiation began to have a serious effect. I haven't had a second bone scan. The rate and extent of decline in my PSA suggest I don't need one. However, as insurance, I'm going to treat all my bones with self-hypnosis to cleanse them of any "normal" cancer cells as well as any radiation-resistant ones that may have escaped the prostate, the seminal vesicles and the lymph nodes.

How to treat bone? By injecting a liquid into the bloodstream, the way the bone scan was done? I imagine an exotic liquid able to differentiate between cancer lesions and arthritic ones, and also able to dissolve the former as if with an acid. But the image of sticking a needle into my vein makes me squeamish. Shall I try radiation? But that would affect my skull, and I dislike the idea of irradiating my brain. (A remembered joke: the trouble with an open mind is that the brain falls out.) So I return to injection, which I've actually experienced and which was "good" for me: it proclaimed (with what certainty I'm unsure) the cancer-free condition of my bones.

I visualize a syringe and its needle. The needle enters a vein of my extended left arm. I feel a comforting liquid being injected. It spreads to my bones. My actual breathing grows slow, steady, deep. A peaceful feeling embraces me. My bones warm up. A nap threatens. "Stay awake," I think, "this is serious business." My raised left arm, tiring, threatens to descend. I count 3, 2, 1 and let it rest on the two pillows. I shut my eyes, roll them upwards gently. I inhale deeply. I count 1, 2, 3, 4, 5 as I exhale, my left arm rising with helium. The session resumes. Now my mind is imageless as the liquid does its work.

Although, as I understand it, X rays with an energy of 15 million electron volts are not likely to be carcinogenic, their penumbras, having lower energies in areas away from the main focus, can be. Major technological efforts are made to diminish the width of the penumbras, yet patients undergoing high-energy therapy may still be exposed to them. As we've seen, they're also potentially exposed to other carcinogenic rays, produced because the 15 MV rays lose some energy through penetrating the patient, and lose still more as they ricochet off the treatment room's walls, floor and ceiling. I've decided to treat such secondary cancers on the off-chance they may exist.

Assuming that the best path is via the immune system, I decide to invent an immune system "control room." Where am I likely to locate such a room? In the brain? But I mistrust the brain, possibly because mammals with brains greatly inferior to our own manage to possess excellent immune systems. In the heart? The heart has enough to do. The adrenals, the two ductless glands (one above each kidney) that power the body when it needs to fight or flee? For reasons obscure yet satisfactory, I'm comfortable with the adrenals though my acquaintance with them is trivial. Question: how to approach them? "Please enrich yourselves with extra blood," I silently say to them, "and send rich blood throughout your immune system to strengthen it. And destroy all secondary cancers, however stray and timid they may appear to be." Visualizing the adrenals, I imagine extra, powerful blood flowing to them.

OCTOBER 30, 1993, MacDowell Colony. A rainy, gloomy afternoon. I drove into Peterborough, the center of which is about a mile from the Colony, for a coffee and a plain, homemade donut at Nonie's on Grove Street and picked up, at Steele's, some color photographs I took at Point Lobos, California. Back in my studio, feeling interior, I face the large fireplace rather than the broad, green-brownish meadow, backed by green trees, beyond my beautiful, many-paned windows. In the old days when I was here, with less creaky knees, I used to delight in making a fire.

Now the fireplace, ready with logs, kindling and a shiny new metal bucket for ashes, leaves me cold. My studio is warm, gracious, almost grand, hinting at a young, Henry Jamesian servant, not me, bending to make and stoke a fire and to gather and dispose of ashes.

I remember, for some reason, the RRS (Royal Research Ship) *Bransfield*, a British Antarctic research ship in the early part of 1977. This was off the Antarctic Peninsula. After the day's work ashore I'd go to the elegant wardroom (tweed jackets, breast-pocket handkerchiefs, liqueurs) and be amused by the artificial fireplace with its winking electric flames. Outdoors were the cold sea, a polar wind, icebergs, pancake ice, brash. I'm reminded of a Santa Cruz friend who proudly showed me his new, outsize bedroom, pulled out a remote control gadget, and with a touch of a button ignited gas flames under artificial fireplace logs.

Moving to the sofa, I start self-hypnosis. I have trouble visualizing my adrenals. They're behind me, as are my kidneys. Solution: I imagine standing a couple of yards from myself and seeing my abstract back, which is neither naked nor clothed. Because I have special vision I can see my outlined kidneys. They resemble supermarket kidneys but are larger, and above each is an adrenal gland. No sweat if this geography is cockamamie; self-hypnosis welcomes making the necessary corrections.

Does it matter that I don't know what the adrenals look like? I doubt it. I sense it's probably counterproductive to insist on being logical in the present context. In my mind's eye they're amorphous twins. I pat them fondly while telling them they're wonderful. They respond by engorging themselves with blood. "Share it," I request. They send blood flowing to the immune system. "If you aren't the system's control room," I say, "I'm sure you know who is. Kindly pass along the message that I need this kind of help." Busily receiving and sending blood, they ignore my comment. The session proceeds peacefully.

OCTOBER 31. A miserable, rainy day, but I'm working well, I don't know why. And I no longer feel lonely here. Matthew Goodman, a writer of short stories, related an anecdote at breakfast. He and his girlfriend, hitchhiking in Maine, were picked up by an old man in a truck. "You used to see a lotta hitchhikers out on the roads. You don't see so many nowadays," the old man said. (Matthew is talented at imitating a Maine accent.) "Why's that?" Matthew asked. "I guess they all got to where they were going," was the reply.

A dull morning, glowering, wet. Silence except for when the heat goes on. No bird sounds except for an occasional cawing. Why is a crow call described as "caw," when actually the sound is "aw"?

My eyes are shut in self-hypnosis. Subject: my urethra, seminal vesicles and lymph nodes. The urethra is a tube that discharges urine from the bladder and semen from the prostate and seminal vesicles. I'll use a ruby laser because, being so vivid and familiar to me, it's easy to visualize. Getting set, I imagine looking down at my groin. My groin recoils; it's too sensitive for a laser attack. I imagine a disembodied penis, urethra and bladder. An improvement, but not good enough. I imagine them on an operating table. Now the laser ranges over the urethra, sweeping it for cancer cells.

I use a green laser for the seminal vesicles. I address my brain. "Pinpoint the seminal vesicles. Direct the green laser at them." The green laser searches for them. The ruby laser handles the urethra. A yellow laser deals with the lymph nodes. I'm treated to a colorful display such as I never had during self-hypnosis for my eyelid, for then I had only one target, and though I used several laser colors, I never did so simultaneously.

Later, thinking, "Where's the harm in experimenting?" I decide to reduce my prostate's size by compression. I imagine a machine, exactly the gland's contours, operated by hydraulic pressure. The machine squeezes the gland. I feel actual discomfort in my groin. The machine continues, and the discomfort threatens to become acute. I return to my original method: reaming out the gland.

NOVEMBER 4. A dull, moody, overcast day, with frost in the morning. Am getting a bit of cabin fever. Last evening, in Colony Hall, a female photographer gave a very powerful presentation with black-and-white projected slides. Subject: her mastectomy. She showed photos of herself nude; and of herself together with her mother, both nude. I was greatly impressed by her bravery and candor. Afterwards there was dancing at the library, a separate building. I observed. One young woman was wonderfully wild and loose in her movements. It's still odd to me to see people dancing singly.

Some thoughts. Is there any point in trying to reduce PSA in itself? Is PSA always just a symptom, not a cause? As I understand it, it's a protein essential to keeping the prostatic part of semen liquid. Why does its population increase dramatically when cancer cells are present? Because cancer cells, like benign ones, work to keep semen from thickening or solidifying? Why does semen solidify? Is PSA a sort of analog to the blood anti-clotting factor? Semen solidifies in air. Does it also solidify in a woman?

Why are prostate cancer cells programmed to do proper semen work; that is, to keep the prostatic semen liquid so it can easily exit the gland? On the one hand these cells help the process of sexual reproduction; on the other they destroy it and, if given the chance, destroy the host as well. Are cancer cells identical with benign cells except in two respects: their ability to replicate rapidly, and to colonize beyond the gland? Is their structural deformity due to overcrowding?

What would happen if you injected benign prostate cells into bone? Would they take root, or would they be destroyed as intruders? What is it in cancer cells that disarms bone? Is the "normal" cancer cell programmed to travel and colonize from the very beginning, and is the one that doesn't travel, the one that produces a low Gleason grade, the timid one, "abnormal"? Why do cancer cells work to prevent semen from thickening and/or solidifying in areas, such as bone, where it's irrelevant whether semen is liquid or not? Or is it not irrelevant? Why should bone care about semen's liquidity? Why is bone friendly to prostate cancer cells? What's in it for bone to harbor cells that will eventually destroy the host?

Has the body's "central control" gone nuts? Is it in some respects "evil," intent on being sadistic, murderous? Species kill other species to survive. Is it possible that in the human body (past a certain age) there is intercellular warfare? Can we inject bone with a substance hostile to prostate cancer cells? Why do such cells have a "preference" for bone? (Why do different cancers have different travel preferences?) Does bone have an active role in prostate cancer metastasis? Does it advertise, "Come to our great, friendly climate"?

Let's say one could, by one means or another (self-hypnosis, for example), inhibit the production of PSA. Would it affect benign cells? Would it change the nature of cancer cells? Would it cause problems with ejaculation (and fertility) because of too-thick semen? Does an excess of PSA cause too-thin semen? Is it possible that PSA is an avenue at getting at the cancer cells?

Why does PSA throw false positives? Is this due to inadequacies in the testing process; or does it indicate a genuine fluctuation in the production of the protein? Is there a central control that says, "Semen is getting too thick. Increase PSA to thin it." Or, "Reduce PSA. The semen has become too thin." Can semen be too thick or too thin? Does a false positive indicate thickening semen? Has anyone done a correlation between semen density and PSA? False positives are alarming, but they do more damage emotionally than physically. False negatives are soothing but dangerous.

PSA rises with the replication of cancer cells because the latter are capable of achieving great populations. Overcrowding causes them to colonize, become imperialistic. They're driven

from within. Which causes the gland to suffer from a deterioration of the quality of life. It's not the gland that first dies, but the
whole empire, which suffers a catastrophic collapse.

Semen volume declines with age, as do sperm population
and the force and intensity of ejaculation. Does semen thicken
with age? And if so, does this mechanism play a role in benign
prostatic hypertrophy? Is the central control (essentially obedi-
ent to the needs of human reproduction) alarmed by the thickening process, and does it take action to reduce the thickening by
calling up cancer cells, with their spectacular ability to increase
PSA (by adding anti-thickening factor to semen)? Suppose we
could invent a chemical, harmless to the human body, able to reduce thickening of semen. Would it have an important effect in
reducing the incidence of prostate cancer?

In normal young men a balance is maintained between the
anti-thickening and the thickening factors in semen. (Is the reduced volume of semen in elderly men partially due to increased thickness, and is ejaculate sluggishness also due to it?)
With age the anti-thickening factor declines in strength. Why?
Is it part of a general "thickening" of the whole body? Cousin
Erik believes prostate cancer is a way of finishing you off because you're no longer useful in sexual reproduction. But if a
boy's prostate is removed, eliminating his ability to reproduce
sexually (at any rate through sexual intercourse), he can't get
prostate cancer. At the height of a male's sexual powers, is
semen in its most liquid form consonant with maximizing his
ability to procreate—the more fluid the semen, the greater the
sperm's motility?

What would happen if one implanted a sample of prostatic
cancer in a female? Would there be something in the female in-
imical to it? Do females possess an anti-prostate factor? Human
males sometimes get breast cancer. Is this cancer similar to
human female breast cancer, or is it very different? Will a sample
of female breast cancer, implanted in a male, produce female
breast cancer? Will it produce male breast cancer? Will it fail to

take root? Is it possible that basically at work here, hidden in the genes, is a model of an androgynous human, and that medical conditions, including disease, are more likely to depend on this model than on a separation of genders? In this sense is there a profound connection between breast cancer and prostate cancer, both of which are currently epidemic in the United States?

NOVEMBER 6. Erik and Molly drove up yesterday to visit me, staying in a Peterborough motel. I spent much of yesterday and today with them, and showed them around the Colony and around the Peterborough environs, such as Hancock, Dublin and Jaffrey. We dined out in Peterborough and Hancock.

NOVEMBER 13. Much frost this morning. The entire large meadow beyond my French doors was gray-white.

A self-hypnosis session. The goal: to lower my PSA. I imagine my brain without its casing of skull. The brain is speaking directly to the prostate's epithelial cells. "Lower the PSA," it's ordering, as if with God's voice. It keeps repeating the sentence. What does it mean to lower the PSA by a direct order? (Lupron, a drug, works by interfering with the brain's orders to the testicles to produce testosterone.) If the brain can order the testicles to produce testosterone, maybe it can also command the prostatic epithelial cells to make cancer. We tend to think of cancer cells as being a kind of mistake. What if they're part of a bodily program? What if the current epidemic of breast and prostate cancers is due to an increased national mental disturbance, an irritation that causes the brain to send negative messages more frequently? Is it possible there's a species population control in the brain?

Sentence fragments and images while I'm half nodding:

"Well, even before you start healing you have to do housekeeping. . . ."

A smiling ancient face, Egyptian, seen in profile. A black cat, walking gingerly toward me, claws outstretched, looking fearful, suddenly leaps to my right.

"You never woke up," said to somebody who apparently was hurt in an accident.

"You wouldn't last clean roots. Your time?"

"No. He can't. He really has a sender of foam with him."

"And what is a nice day? For a moment? No, for self-hypocrisy. You called Io a Geo. A Geo is. . . ."

"The roof of summer coming over."

"You have any? Ask for it! You don't want to do the rabbi!"

"If you're hammering . . . that's the time to begin."

"He was incapable of being thrown off a horse, and under a sycamore."

"I ask you to warn, your life insurance has given up."

"Missa Neagle is both a horse."

"Guess where the other penis is. The extra affair."

"We got three-quarters of the afternoon registered, and she said, 'Mesmerate.'"

"They're making affairs all over this country, and the fondue spirit is all suffragism."

NOVEMBER 26, 1993, MACDOWELL COLONY. At times I feel I'm ready to leave here for the real world. A number of us began playing poker last week, and have continued playing quite frequently. I joined the game on condition that we banish wild cards.

Kate Doyle called from Santa Cruz last evening to report that she went to the Newtown cancer support group meeting on Wednesday. Lois's husband, Jimmy, is still alive. Sheila (lung cancer that metastasized to her brain) is doing well. So is Wendy (Hodgkin's disease). Brigid (ovarian cancer) no longer wears a turban. Patty (the "newcomer") is getting chemotherapy and has lost her hair. Kate didn't chat at any length with Henry Trout, but she learned he's on Lupron and is still considering having cryosurgery. Sandra's husband, Luke (metastasized squamous cell carcinoma), is close to death.

Bunny and Lloyd were both at the meeting. Lloyd (liver and pancreatic cancer) was in the hospital recently, and Sandra thought he had only a week or two more of life, but she was wrong. He looks more gaunt and tired. Bunny and Lloyd will soon have their twenty-fifth wedding anniversary but lack the money to celebrate it.

Sandra said, "We're so po' we can't afford the *r*."

Brigid said, "I'm so poor I can't even pay attention."

People remarked on how cancer has brought good things to them; shown them how to cherish life.

"Thanks, oh Lord, for the thorn in my side," somebody said.

How remarkable that science has instruments capable of detecting weights as fine as billionths of a gram. My last PSA of 6.2 means there were 6.2 billionths of a gram of the antigen per thousandth of a liter of my blood.

It will be interesting to see what my PSA will be early in January. Will it remain at 6.2, my last reading? Will it dip a bit, maybe go down to 5.8? Will it start to rise?

Thirteen

December 10, 1993, to February 4, 1994

DECEMBER 10, 1993, MACDOWELL COLONY. Until the other day, specifically about 2:00 P.M. of December 8, I had never had a car accident although I'm almost seventy-nine and obtained my first driver's license at the age of thirteen. That was in 1928 in Richmond, Virginia, when my car was a used Overland my father had bought for me for $25. I seem to remember the Overland's vintage was 1925, but I must be mistaken, the car couldn't possibly have been only three years old. Its tires were so thin they sometimes got caught in streetcar tracks. (Richmond had many trolley lines in those days.) It had brakes on the rear wheels only. I'd adjust them with a pair of pliers before a trip, and sometimes during one.

In highway traffic when a line of cars ahead of me came to a stop I'd have a minor heart attack as the Overland would slow down ever so slowly, no matter how hard and far I pressed on the brake pedal. (The emergency brake was almost useless.) Despite the fact that I tried to keep a long distance between me and the car ahead, it always felt like a miracle that the Overland came to a stop just in time. It was a temperamental car. Sometimes smoke issued from under the dashboard. I paid little attention to this until on one occasion the dashboard burst into flames from an electrical fire. That was the beginning of the end of my love affair with that car.

Anyhow, up until the accident the other day, I was having a pleasant afternoon car excursion. My passenger was Shirley Most, a middle-aged painter, who had never been to Jaffrey or Rindge or Fitzwilliam, New Hampshire towns in the vicinity of Peterborough. I took her first to Jaffrey, where she bought some things at a thrift shop. Then we went to Jaffrey Center, a beautiful village with a lovely old church. Behind the church are a number of restored horse stalls, some going back to 1810. Behind these is the cemetery where Willa Cather was buried. It has been a tradition for colonists to visit her grave. But I couldn't locate it, I don't know why.

Then we headed toward Fitzwilliam because I wanted to show Shirley the charming village and its common, and nearby Laurel Lake, where my wife, Joan, used to go to Fleur de Lis Camp as a girl. We took 202 south from Jaffrey, went west on 119 and came to an intersection with 12. 119 had a blinking red light. 12 had a blinking amber one. I came to a dead stop. Looking in both directions, we didn't see any cars. I began crossing the highway.

What I remember most vividly now, two days after the accident, is that a sudden darkness descended on my window, an occlusion of light, while simultaneously I heard the wild, unbelievable crushing of metal, *my* metal, and sensed flying objects outside my car. There was no warning whatever, no honk of a horn, no screeching of tires. The collision came randomly out of the blue, like a meteor or a cancer, both potentially fatal. I thought, "I'm having a car accident, the first in my life, and this scratch-free, wonderful Camry is being crushed."

We spun to the right. We had our seat belts on; we weren't flung anywhere. I hit the brake, put the car in park, got out and walked around. Most of my car's left side was undamaged, but its left front had been ripped open. Pieces were hanging there, some of them wires. Other pieces were on the highway. There were no skid marks. My left front tire had blown out. Its wheel had been wrecked. A large pickup truck, having made a 180-degree turn, was facing my car. There was a long black gash in the upper part of its right front tire, which had blown out, and some minor damage to the right fender. The driver climbed out of the truck.

I said, "I came to a dead stop. Where'd you come from? You hit me!"

"They all say that," he said, grinning.

A man came out of the filling-station store at the junction.

"Call the cops," I said.

"They're on their way," he replied.

Moving around, I felt uninjured. I poked my head into the Camry and asked, "Are you okay?"

"My head hurts, and my back hurts," said Shirley Most.

Two young cops arrived in a Fitzwilliam cruiser. A fire engine, an ambulance and several private cars converged on the scene. Some of the firemen wore orange suits. Shirley, having been trussed in a neck collar and back brace, was carried to a stretcher and driven away in the ambulance.

Somebody aimed the beam of a pencil flashlight into my eyes and ears. Men kept asking if I was okay. I said I felt fine. They brought out a folding chair they asked me to sit on, then fitted me out the way they had done Shirley. Someone squatting in front of me, with long brown nostril hair, said if the pickup truck had hit me two feet further back I probably would have been killed. Sitting close behind the fire engine, I was breathing its exhaust fumes. When I mentioned this, the man turned the engine off. Don Bailey, of Bailey's Garage in Fitzwilliam, towed my car away.

An ambulance came from Winchenden, Massachusetts, and took me to Monadnock Community Hospital in Peterborough, where Shirley's back was being X-rayed. The ride in the ambulance, my first, was unpleasant. The stretcher was cold and kept swaying, especially when we took curves. It reminded me of being on an icebreaker on the Southern Ocean. The emergency room doctor found nothing wrong with

Shirley's X rays. He gave her two prescriptions, one for Flexeril (cyclobenzaprine), a muscle relaxant, the other for a strong pain killer, probably containing codeine. She filled only the Flexeril. He found me to be all right.

I felt spooked for two or three days after the accident. The adrenaline rush had left hormonal imbalance in its wake. Both my mind and my body told me they needed time to return to normal. A couple of colonists asked me if I'd feel anxious about driving again. I said I didn't know. I recalled a helicopter pilot asking me in Antarctica, a day or so after I had crashed in a helicopter near the summit of Mount Erebus, if I was willing to fly again, because the skipper of an icebreaker wanted me to join him for dinner on the ship, which was in McMurdo Sound. Smiling, I had said, "No problem. I love flying in helicopters." Would I feel the same way when I got behind the wheel of my car?

DECEMBER 22. My car was repaired very satisfactorily in Fitzwilliam, New Hampshire, and I wasn't gun-shy about driving it again. I left the MacDowell Colony the morning of the 21st after a stay of two months and drove to Cousin Erik's in Irvington, New York. Erik said he had a new experience with Dr. Fledermaus, his urologist, to share with me. The following is his account.

I see Fledermaus twice a year, mainly to check my PSA. I'd have a problem if it were anything above 0.00, because it would mean the cancer had spread. Before December 10 I had been building up a head of steam. I felt I should reveal my anger to him because he had cut the erectile nerves. But then I thought, "What the hell, it's all done, what's the point of giving it to him?" So my relationship has been hearty, outgoing. On simple procedures such as follow-ups, I still see him, but I would never allow him to operate on me again. During my last visit, on December 10, he asked a number of questions about my health. Then he got into my sex life. I said, "It's nil."

He asked, "What about the vacuum method?"

"It's no good," I said, "at least for me. It's too painful. Also, the constriction of the rubber bands at the base of the penis makes it difficult to penetrate, because the penis doesn't have a base, it flaps in the wind. I'm capable of a semi-erection, but not enough for penetration."

He said, "What you should do is masturbate as frequently as possible to keep the muscles active and the rhythms going."

I said, "I haven't experienced ejaculation."

He said, "You can expect only urine to come out of your penis, because I tied off the tubes. If you have an orgasm, what you'll be getting is a sensation in your brain. The brain is the true source of an orgasm. But for you, ejaculation isn't possible. What about trying the self-injection method?"

He showed me a needle and said it's the kind used by diabetes patients who inject themselves with insulin. The injection is made at a right angle into the shaft of the penis, where the erectile tubes are. In ten or fifteen minutes you begin getting an erection, which lasts about an hour. He cautioned that if I use too much of the drug and my penis remains erect for a period of four hours, I'll have to go to the emergency room of a hospital to get another injection into my penis to counteract the drug, or I'll have to go to his office to have it done. He said that does sometimes happen.

I said, "Sticking a needle into my penis is not what I consider fun."

He said, "I've had a lot of success with a number of patients, although one patient who was able to function with the method stopped using it, I don't know why. It's a fairly easy procedure. If you decide to try it you'll have to see me three times so I can teach you how to self-inject; also so I can determine the exact amount of the drug needed to give you an erection." He gave me some literature about the method. "Read it carefully," he said. "You'll have to sign a consent form."

In reading the literature, I was alarmed by the possible side effects. This is a fairly new method, and the doctors know little about the potential long-term damage. There are many things that can happen. For example, if you have a swollen or black-and-blue penis, you have to compress the whole penis with your hand for ten minutes. This should *prevent further swelling. I'm sure my partner would be very interested in a two-tone penis. The needle may cause bleeding in the blood vessels. If it's inserted too high, it can injure penile nerves and arteries or veins. If it's inserted too low, it can injure the urethra. It can cause penile skin irritation; scarring of the erectile tissue; infection of the skin; injury to the artery of the erectile tissue; changes in heart rhythm; liver injury. It's essential, beforehand, to have a blood count and an electrocardiogram, because in some rare cases the drug has caused strokes. You must maintain strict sterile technique. Also, it's essential to have monthly follow-ups, which include blood tests and a cardiogram.*

He said the method isn't painful, but I don't think having sex this way makes sense for me. Sex is supposed to be a pleasant experience. In the back of my head I'd be waiting for a stroke to happen.

DECEMBER 29, 1993, PRINCETON, NEW JERSEY. Even though I'm doing well, such is the nature of cancer that I'm in some suspense regarding my next PSA. I think Dr. North believes it will be at least as low as my last one, 6.2. Why do I rather expect it to have risen a bit?

I phoned Henry Lombardi of the support group to arrange to interview him. When I asked how he's doing, he replied, "Fine. I've been lucky." An interesting response from someone who's impotent as a consequence of a prostatectomy and hormone therapy. Again it brings to mind the relativity of having cancer. All of us in the support group are in the same odd boat. No, we're in different little boats, but in the same rapidly flowing river, with its special shoals.

JANUARY 3, 1994. I interviewed Lombardi this afternoon in the living room of his King City house. Only Henry and I were present. He's sixty-six, has thick white carefully groomed hair, and looks to be in good shape despite a modest abdominal bulge. He wore an old brown plaid woolen shirt buttoned up to the throat, and scuffed brown shoes. His small teeth resemble a child's when he smiles or laughs. The skin on his roundish face is loose and a bit wrinkly. His voice is muffled, soft, shy.

"How and when did you discover you have prostate cancer?" I began.

I was due for a physical, and I made arrangements with my doctor to have one. I have one every two years. He noticed that my prostate gland was a little hard, so he suggested that I see a urologist. He also said, "I want to take one more sample of blood." When the test, a PSA, came back, he says, "Your PSA is 53." And he says, "You want to get to a urologist right away. Let him check you out and see if he confirms my findings."

This was two and a half years ago. That was Dr. Pomeroy. Then I went to Dr. Gilroy. And Gilroy says, "Well, we'll run some tests." He did the ultrasound, and he said, "I'm pretty positive that you've got cancer, but we need a biopsy to make sure. If you want to, we can do it right now."

I said, "Okay." So he took seven samples, and later five showed traces of cancer. It was an unpleasant procedure, but better than I expected. [Lombardi made a wry face.] *He told me the needle travels at fifty miles an hour. It goes right in and right out.*

This was in May 1991. I was sixty-four, and feeling pretty good. The Gleason reading was 6, so Gilroy gave me my options. He says, "You could have the radical operation, or you could have radiation. The trouble with radiation is, it's good for maybe four to six years, and the operation is good for ten or twelve."

So I says, "Well, if I do anything, I'll go for the ten or twelve." But I said, "I also want to have a second opinion."

I decided I would contact a friend of mine down at the University of Pennsylvania. He's a urologist, and he teaches there. His father and I are very good friends. So he told me to come down, and that he had a very good urologist there, a young fellow. He introduced me to him, and that was Dr. Steven Horowitz.

I asked Horowitz, I says, "How many operations do you do like this every year?"

He says, "Between me and my partner about a hundred and fifty."

And Dr. Gilroy told me he does about twelve. So I says to my-self, "I'd be a lot better off having somebody who does it all the time, who knows exactly what he's looking for, and has new ideas, a young fellow."

My wife and daughter went down there with me, and they agreed that I should go to the University of Pennsylvania. Dr. Horowitz is thirty-eight. When I saw his resume I was really shocked. Because he was at the University of Vermont the same time that my daughter was. Same years and everything, but different fields. My daughter was an art major. I think you've got to have young doctors today. Because they're up-to-date on all the newest things, new equipment, and all that stuff. I feel sorry for the older doctors. After a certain period of time they can't keep up with everything. Horowitz did my prostatectomy. I go to him every six months for a PSA now.

But what happened was, my wife had a heart attack and she needed a triple bypass. So I decided I would wait for my operation, because my cancer doesn't grow that fast, and let my wife go in and have her oper-ation. She went at the end of June. She came out on a Saturday and I went in the next day. My daughters were home to take care of my wife, and they thought it was best if I went as soon as possible. That way we'd both be convalescent together, since my daughters were taking time off to take care of us.

The only thing that happened was—you know that after the oper-ation you have a catheter. And I had the catheter in for a day and a half. And then something happened. I couldn't urinate. I told the resident, and the resident brought the other doctors, and they called Horowitz up, and Horowitz said, "The balloon must have broken on the end of the catheter." He says, "I'll be in very soon."

It was probably about 9:30 at night. In an hour he was there. He took me down to the X-ray room, and the X rays showed that the bal-loon did break and was blocking the urine from coming out. He says, "I hate to do this to you, but we've got to, we've got to change the catheter." So they pulled the catheter out and put another one in. But that was the only problem.

When they do that operation they check the lymph nodes first, and if there's any cancer in the lymph nodes they stop the operation. There was no cancer showing in my lymph nodes in the operating room. They sent seventeen lymph nodes out to a lab to check. When they got the results a couple of weeks later, they found that there were cancer cells in one lymph node. So Horowitz suggested that I have radiation and go on hormone therapy. He says, "I want you to talk to the radiologist too."

I talked to the radiologist, and the radiologist says, "If it was me, I'd have radiation. Instead of you coming back here every day, you have a real good radiology department in King City. I trained two of those people up there."

So I says, "Okay."

I had thirty-six treatments. But it was a lighter treatment than if you didn't have the operation. It didn't bother me a bit. I was a little tired, but that's about all.

And I was doing hormone therapy at the same time. I was getting an injection of Lupron once a month. And I take six Eulexin pills a day, two every eight hours, around the clock. Lupron and Eulexin are chemical castration. They told me I would be on them the rest of my life. The thing with the hormone therapy is, you have a tendency to wear off after forty-two months, they say. When Dr. Horowitz first put me on this, he says, "You're better off going with this, and in the meantime we might find something better." I was talking with him about this the last time I saw him, and he said they're finding out it lasts longer than forty-two months.

Lupron works on a twenty-eight-day cycle. They want you to get a shot every twenty-eight days. They give you the shot in the buttocks, and that's it. The only problem is, it's very expensive. It's $485 for the shot. And then they charge you $35 to give it to you. But Medicare takes care of it. It's ridiculous to charge you $35 to give you the shot. Because I can go in there and be out in less than five minutes.

Horowitz says, "You've done very well."

I asked him the last time, I says, "How about if I go off the hormone therapy?"

He says, "I wouldn't do that yet." He says, "Even though there's no reading on your PSA, I would stay on that for a while yet."

And I says, "Well, how about my sex life?" I said, "I would like to regain that."

He says, "Well, maybe we can do something else about that. But I would stay on the hormone therapy."

So I figured I would just stay on it and see what happens after maybe another couple of years.

I get the hot flashes. I still get anywhere from six to eight a day. In my case I think it's going to continue, because usually by this time they start to fall off. They're not that bad. They last a few minutes. But you get real hot. Sometimes the sweat will roll off my face. My PSA is 0.0. It's lasted for two and a half years so far.

"Did you have any trouble accepting the diagnosis of prostate cancer?" I asked.

I was in good condition when I found out about it. It came as a shock to me. I had no problems. I knew my sex life wasn't what it was ten years ago, but I expected that. Every once in a while, when I'd go to urinate, it would be a little slower than normal, but that's part of aging too. If I hadn't gone for my physical I wouldn't have known anything about it. But no, I had no problem accepting the diagnosis. The doctors are there to help me, not to hurt me. And if I've got this, I've got to learn to live with it. I'm dealt this hand and I've got to play it out. And you've got to go at it with a positive outlook.

My wife took it harder than I did.

When we went to see Dr. Gilroy to get the final report, and he showed us all the X rays and everything, and the bone scan and the CAT scan, and all that, he put them up on the screen, and he was talking about all these hot spots, and my wife says, "I can't believe that."

Well, these hot spots were arthritis, but he didn't say that right at the beginning. He shocked the daylights out of my wife.

And then she says, "Is that all cancer?"

And he says, "No, it's arthritis."

"Have you looked into any methods of dealing with impotence?"

I went to a meeting at King City Hospital. They were having a seminar one night, and my wife and I went to that. And they talked about doing implants. And they passed the silicone implants around. And they had a pump, to give me an erection. I talked to Horowitz about that. And he says, "Well, if you decide to do that, come and talk to us about it." I said, "Right now I don't want to do anything."

But I think maybe I should do something, because I think it creates a lot of frustration in my wife. I think she gets frustrated. She's always trying to do something all the time. She keeps herself busy all the time. Of course, she's always been like this, but since my operation she's done more of it. So there's frustration there, there's no doubt of it. And there's frustration on my part. She says, "You had a lot of patience before, but now you don't have that much."

And I think this is a real mistake we make, by not talking about it. At the support meeting, I think we should talk more about it. And I think that even in our own education as we grow up over the years we don't talk enough about it. It's something you're going to do every day of your life the rest of your life, and nobody tells you anything about it. They teach us everything else in school, but they don't teach us anything about what we're going to do every day in our life.

I hope the fellows in the support group will speak frankly about it. That's why I keep bringing it up every once in a while, to see what reactions I get from them. I want to see what their feelings are, compared to mine. And if the women are there, the women are just as interested as we are.

Well, my wife and I have had a pretty good life together. She accepts that I'm impotent. And we feel, well, we've got each other. And that counts. And we have four very good children that we never had any problems with, and that makes a big difference.

I think it's very valuable to belong to a support group. The more you talk about a problem you have, the easier it is to live with it. And you learn from other people. And if you talk about a subject, you're going to be more at ease, you're going to find out what's best to do and what's not. I don't think men should worry so much about the loss of sex life as they do, because you can still have a good life without it. I think too many men worry about that. And that's why they hesitate to have it taken care of. And then it's too late. And men don't want to talk about it.

I have friends who have prostate cancer who won't come to the meetings, they don't want to talk about it. There's one fellow here, a business man, he has a pretty successful business, and he's had prostate cancer for about eight years, and I tried to get him to come and join the group. He's got time to do it. He says, "No, I don't want to be involved with it." He comes to King City to get his Lupron shot every month. And he says, "You know, you go to those groups," and he says, "You meet the fellows, and a couple months later they're gone." He says, "I don't want that."

That's what these fellows think. Just because you're in a support group, you're on your last legs. And that's not true. I think that the main thing about prostate cancer is that we're getting more publicity about it now. More people are becoming aware of it. I think the more men hear about it, the more men talk about it, the better off they are. I've had people come up to me, and they would hesitate to talk to me. Especially anything about cancer. And that I think is wrong. I think the more we talk about it ourselves, the more comfortable other people are going to be about it. And they learn from us talking about it. And I don't hesitate to talk about it to anybody.

And I have some brothers and sisters, and a couple of them think I'm an invalid. And I says, "No. Don't define me as an invalid. I'm just as healthy as you are. Don't worry about it." That's when some people look at you, because you have cancer. The breast people are well organized. They've got the money for research, and everything, and I think this is what we've got to do. Because there isn't a big difference between the number of people who die from prostate cancer and the number of people who die from breast cancer. We're all statistics coming out.

JANUARY 4, 1994. Today is exactly seven months since I finished radiation therapy. There was a sleet storm all last night and this morning. The yew bushes in front of the house are a massive, sparkling ice sculpture, full of diamonds sporting tiny rainbows. I had blood drawn for a PSA this afternoon. Will the new PSA be a good omen? A bad one? It would be extraordinary to go below 4, and nice to go below 5, but I'd be content with a repeat of mid-October's 6.2, which in some people's opinion is within the upper limit of normal for my age. Also, before therapy I had a very large gland, and presumably still have one, and that should raise the PSA a bit.

Shall I make a guess at a figure? I'll say 5.8.

JANUARY 6, THURSDAY. I got a call this morning from Dr. North, who said excitedly, "I have your new PSA! Take a number."

"5.8."

"4.0! It may go even lower! It's a *very* dramatic change! We'll discuss it on Monday."

Ten years ago we hadn't heard of a PSA test. Now so much depends on it.

JANUARY 8, SATURDAY. I called Henry Trout in Newtown today. "I understand you're on hormone therapy," I said.

"Right."

"What's your PSA?"

"7.1."

"Has the Lupron affected you sexually?"

"Big time. Especially the ejaculation. It's like when you're about to sneeze, and somebody is squeezing your nose, and has a headlock on you, and you sneeze anyway. That's how you ejaculate—like a ladyfinger firecracker."

I joined him in a laugh.

"What does Dr. Morgan think about how you're doing?" I asked.

"He still thinks cryosurgery is questionable. Too experimental. We'll talk to Harkin. And collect more facts. And there's an outfit in Bethesda, Maryland, I want to get some facts from. How's your weather?"

"11 degrees this morning. And it snowed last night, on top of lots of ice. How's yours?"

"Balmy, like spring. Things are turning green."

Kate Doyle called from Santa Cruz to say she attended the Newtown support group on Wednesday. Sandra's husband, Luke (squamous cell carcinoma), has died. So have Lois's husband, Jimmy (lung cancer), and Maury (pancreatic cancer). I remembered Luke well: killer mustache, shoulder-length hair, brown boots. . . . I had never met Jimmy. I recalled his wife, Lois, talking about waiting for him to die. Had she and her daughter reunited, let go of their grievances? . . . I remembered Maury, whose leanness, deep voice and measured way of speaking had reminded me of my friend Norman Bloomfield, who had died of leukemia. . . .

What strange differences in destiny we mortals have, I thought. Here I am, about to turn seventy-nine, and I seem to be in remission. And there those other guys are . . . or were. . . . What to make of it? Nothing. . . . And I thought of George Henry, of the King City support group, who had recently died a very hard death, according to Harry Stengel. I hadn't known him either. Try not to feel guilty, I told myself. Try to just let it be. Accept the inevitable. Much easier said than done.

JANUARY 10, 1994. I had a follow-up visit with Dr. North this morning. As usual, he wore a white coat. He looked happy and youthful. "How are you feeling?" he asked.

"Fine. My urine stream seems much stronger."

"How often do you wake up at night?"

"Once or twice. Also, I retain urine longer, so when I do go, there's a considerable stream."

"No problems with dribbling or leaking?"

"No. I don't think I ever had that. The only side effect I now have, aside from this good one of a better stream, is in my gait.

If I'm walking my normal power walk I don't feel it. When I get out of the car and stroll to a supermarket, sometimes I have a kind of rolling gait."

"Do you lean to one side or the other? There's not a tendency, for example, to always stumble to the right?"

"There's no stumbling."

"Do you have any pain when you have a bowel movement?"

"No."

"Any blood?"

"No. By the way, what's my acid phosphatase as of January 3?"

"2.3."

I showed him a graph I had drawn of my PSA and acid phosphatase readings, beginning with those at the start of therapy.

"I'm mystified by my 4.0 PSA," I said. "I'm very happy with it, of course, but I'm also puzzled. I don't understand why it's so low. What happened to the model of a gland with an elevated PSA due to benign enlargement? On what basis did you so boldly predict a PSA as low as 4.5 back in October?"

"Like you, I graphed your readings. And then I extrapolated. I'm not as surprised as you are. Your PSA may go even lower than 4.0. I wouldn't be surprised if it tapers off at 3.0."

"Can the prostate have shrunk, causing less pressure on the urethra? If it has shrunk, what part of it is due to the destruction of cancer cells and what part to the destruction of benign ones? It would seem to me there are two scenarios. One, that I had cancer all along but it wasn't detectable; that the early high PSAs—10, 11, 12, 12.5—were due to cancer. And now that the cancer cells are being destroyed, the PSA is coming down. Or, there was a conjunction of the destruction of cancer cells and benign ones. What's your guess as to what's going on?"

"I don't think that all of your cancer cells produced your initial elevation. I think some of it was BPH, benign enlargement, but I can't possibly tell you to what extent. You may have had the cancer for years. It's like sticking your hand into a haystack and trying to find the needle. If you don't have some method of X-raying the haystack and seeing where the needle is, in which quadrant, you're never going to find it. It's very encouraging, though, that your PSA is as low as it is. You're looking for an answer to a puzzle where the final pieces of the puzzle haven't been cut out yet. I don't think anyone has a real good handle on PSA's response yet. I mean, we have our own database from our own experiences. There's lots and lots of follow-up on people now. We've only been using PSA for several years. We don't have ten-year follow-up data on PSA. I've seen a couple of people's PSA drop, and then come back up again to a level which I would have called a BPH level. And there it hovers, and there it stays. And that may just be that there's a temporary suppression of PSA from benign cells, and as they recover slowly over time, they produce a little more PSA. And that's why I don't want you to be alarmed if your PSA does go up to 6 or 7. If it hovers there, then maybe that is what your normal prostate volume is producing, if there's been a temporary suppression of the normal PSA manufactured."

"Let's assume that cancer cells didn't constitute a significant portion of the gland's volume. If this is correct, do you suppose enough benign cells were killed to reduce the gland's size?"

"It's the same question mark. We don't know."

He now gave me a digital exam. I felt his finger probing aggressively, going higher and higher. "The gland feels normal," he said. "I think it's smaller. There's almost no sign of the protuberance. Maybe a trace of scarring. Consistency of the gland is rubbery, good."

He had taken a fecal smear to check for occult blood. Result: negative.

As always, it had been a pleasure to meet with him.

FEBRUARY 4, 1994. I met with my urologist, Dr. Lew Gilroy, today. He asked a number of questions. How's your stream? Pain in urinating? Any difficulty? Any blood? Bowel movements normal? Any blood? Unusual backaches? Although the prostate is a sexual organ, he asked no sexual questions. At his request, I dropped my trousers and undershorts and lay on my back on a gurney. He examined my penis and testicles, then palpated my abdomen and groin, asking if there was any pain. While I sat on the gurney's end he pummeled my lower back, again asking if there was pain. I assumed he was looking for signs of bone metastases. He didn't seem surprised by my 4.0 PSA.

"We didn't tell you," he said, "but if the PSA doesn't drop to 4 by a year after radiation, we suspect the radiation failed."

"What about the effect of benign enlargement on PSA?"

After a long pause he said, "If your PSA goes up to 6 or 6.5, we'll have to wonder if it's due to benign enlargement or to a failure of the radiation."

He did what felt like a prolonged, muscular digital.

"Your gland has shrunk by about 30 percent," he said. "That's good. Probably what has happened is that the blood vessels feeding the benign cells have been damaged by the radiation, and so some cells have died for lack of nourishment. I'd like to see you twice more at intervals of three months. After that, twice a year."

It seemed to me he was not as enthusiastic about my progress as Dr. North. I thought, "Well, he's a surgeon, he sees life from the scalpel's point of view, so it's not surprising he's skeptical about the relative value of radiation."

Fourteen

February 24 to February 25, 1994

FEBRUARY 24, 1994. When I dined in a Manhattan restaurant last week with Dr. Paul Gross, my New York dermatologist friend, I was startled to learn he had never had either a PSA or a DRE (digital rectal exam). I asked if he was willing to talk about that in some detail. He agreed, so we had the following chat in his apartment on lower Fifth Avenue.

We sat on a sofa facing an elegant coffee table. On the table were some pieces of amber (he's interested in insects embalmed in amber), including a polished pendant he said was Baltic amber that had come from Russia (scratched on the back were three Cyrillic initials) and which contained, according to him, a potato beetle among bits of vegetation. He's sixty, small, lean, sensitive, intelligent, cultured.

"Many Americans have become almost idolatrous about the PSA," I said. "Why are you skeptical about it?"

"I'm not skeptical about the PSA per se . . . or only. For myself, I observe a kind of medicine which is not what many doctors preach today [he laughed] . . . or practice . . . and that is, I rarely consult doctors, and I do so only when I think I have something I need an opinion about. I tend to treat myself for minor things, or even fairly discomforting ones if I feel I know what they are and what can be done about them. I have a great deal of confidence in the way I live, and in my genetic heritage.

I believe I'm endowed with basically good health. And I don't feel anxious about my health. And so I don't want to entrust my health to something I don't understand, and I can't understand the PSA. I don't know exactly how it's done. I don't know who'll do it. I don't know what their concentration will be while they're doing it. And I can't account for all the myriad things that may go wrong. I don't think I'm going to get, in this case, cancer of the prostate, and so I don't think I need to have a PSA, which might alarm me and lead to all kinds of tests and biopsies and put me on some kind of circuit where I would lose control."

"Do you have a similar reaction to cholesterol tests?"

"Yes."

"Is there any case where you deviate from this pattern of skepticism?"

"Well, I know a little bit about cholesterol, and I think we don't understand the relationship between the cardiovascular system, longevity and cholesterol. My mother, for example, has a very high cholesterol, and she's 85, and she's still winning dancing contests. She's very neurotic about her cholesterol. She's been taking a drug for the past ten or fifteen years to artificially lower it, because the numbers worry her."

He laughed.

"What's her number?" I asked.

"350."

"I've heard a doctor say the drug that reduces cholesterol may merely reduce cholesterol and not the deposit of plaque."

"I expect it does something like that. But it makes people feel better if they get caught up in the numbers. She has an anxious component to her personality. People tell me horror stories—and I know that some of them are true—because individuals have ignored their cholesterol or their PSA. But one has to choose some kind of ground in life on which to stand."

"Has your mother been athletic all her life?"

"Not athletic at all. Just dancing and walking."

"She dances vigorously now?"

"Social dancing. Fox-trot, waltz, those kinds of things. She loves to do that."

"I assume you haven't had a father or a brother with prostate cancer."

"True. My father would be alive today if he hadn't been addicted to nicotine. He smoked Bull Durham's, the roll-your-own thing, from the time he was twelve, and he developed cancer of the lungs, and was seventy when he died."

He picked up the amber pendant, which was attached to a silver chain, and stroked it.

"It looks too good to be true," I remarked.

"I know."

"Is it possible it's a phony?"

"I suppose it is. But the shop that sold it to me has a good reputation, and assured me it's authentic. Also, I've tested it with a hot needle, and it gave off a strong resin aroma."

"Do you regard colleagues of yours as being eccentric if they pay attention to the PSA?"

"Well, if a patient comes to you and says, 'I want you to examine me' . . . if the patient entrusts himself to you, and you're a medicine man, you're not a shaman . . . you have to use the best knowledge and tools at your command. You're charged with doing the best you can to assure this person that he or she doesn't have a cancer."

"You're not impressed or alarmed by the increasing incidence of prostate cancer? The detection of it has certainly increased."

"I don't know what some of these things mean. In my own field, I'm not sure that there's a real epidemic of skin cancer. We screen more people."

"What about the fact that some medical institutions are recommending that men over forty-five get an annual PSA?"

"They also say you should have a colonoscopy, and I haven't done that either. It's a lot to go through. I had one long ago. The doctor that talked me into it said, 'You don't have to do the whole prep.'" Paul Gross laughed. "If you don't do the whole prep, the doctor can't see very well, and yet the whole prep . . . it knocks you out. It's very onerous to do it. And so, again, you have to weigh how much you want to invest in these things. What I *do* do. . . . I have *some* apprehension about things like bowel cancer, which is fairly common—my mother had a bout with that—so I do do that, I do check my stool once a year. The test is not perfect, but it's easy to do. If you get a false positive, you just do it a couple more times. If you get a false negative, well, it's too bad."

"What about the digital rectal exam?"

"I told myself I should get that—it's a simple thing—when I got to be a certain age . . . when I consulted doctors. But I've never consulted doctors very much. At the various times when I *have* consulted a doctor, they never offered to do it. I didn't ask them to do it, and they never offered to do it. Which is contrary to what we're taught in medical school."

"Were you getting an annual physical?"

"No, I was consulting a doctor about something else. When I *had* physicals they were more or less short, quick ones. Fairly perfunctory. I would have submitted to a digital rectal exam, I guess, if the doctor had said I should have one."

"Do you believe, now, that it's correct to have a DRE once a year?"

"It's a simple enough part of an exam. I don't think you need to do it with people who are twenty or thirty, but with older people it's probably a reasonable thing to do."

"Some Europeans are horrified that we Americans are doing so much with the PSA."

"Yes, we tend to do that. We tend to worship numbers."

"But inasmuch as we don't know the cause of prostate cancer, do you feel any apprehension about not checking your prostate every year?"

"No, I don't have much apprehension about that."

"At dinner you said you think you won't die of prostate cancer, but that you may die of cardiovascular disease."

"I meant by that, dying of old age. In other words, we sort of deteriorate. The system deteriorates, and where it is most in evidence is in the heart and in the brain."

"Obviously there are very good genes on your mother's side."

"My grandmother died of an infectious disease. She was born in the Old World and came here and died of tuberculosis. My maternal grandfather lived into his eighties. He was very active. I don't know what he died of. He knew he was going to die. It was quite remarkable, because he wrote out how everything was to be done, and how the estate was to be divided."

"He wasn't obviously ill?"

"Not to me. He didn't communicate well to me. He spoke mostly Hebrew and Yiddish, and only a little English. I don't think anybody knows what he died of."

"His forebears were from a Slavic country?"

"Russia. Near Odessa. At least, that was their port of exit."

"Is there anybody close to you who's concerned because you're not taking the conventional course in this prostate matter?"

"I don't think so. I don't think anybody—." He laughed. "I can think of all the myriad things that people get apprehensive about. I think that's more attributable to the way the human mind works than to anything else. My mother would get apprehensive about something that she thought I should have checked because she had read about it in the paper. And so will Blanche [his wife] react that way. But that's kind of reacting after the fact."

"Wouldn't it be safer to have your prostate checked in the usual manner? You have car insurance, house insurance. . . ."

"The usual manner being what?"

"Going for a PSA and a DRE."

"It probably would, but the problem is that once you do that, then it's hard to back out of it. If I get an elevated PSA and the doctor doesn't feel anything, he may say, 'Well, you have to have a biopsy.' And an ultrasound. And you start doing all this business. Of course, I could be caught short, I could make a mistake. I realize that, but I just feel I'm not going to be afflicted by prostate cancer. It has to do, I guess, with something you yourself said—that you want to live, but you want to live a certain way. I'm in good health, and I haven't been troubled by anything except the afflictions of old age and a mysterious allergy, and I haven't troubled my colleagues, and I haven't had a lot of laboratory tests and procedures that have taken my time and bothered me."

He put the beautiful amber pendant back on the table.

"Suppose you were looking at somebody close to you. Would you take the same view?" I asked.

"It's very hard. It's very painful. I'll tell you what happened to my father. He felt fine. He went for a routine physical, and he had a routine chest X ray, and they saw a spot on his lung, and he wanted me to help him. He said, 'What should I do?' And I told him to do what the doctor said. And so it involved a biopsy—an exploratory—and the removal of a lung. And he only had a year to live, and so he spent six months being sick and recovering from procedures, and the other six months dying from the disease. If he hadn't done anything, he would have had six months more to live. How do you advise somebody? It seems foolish not to take advantage of medical procedures and medical training, but sometimes they really don't avail anything, and are counterproductive to the life span of the individual. I think if you enjoy good health and you don't have a family history of certain diseases, you have a pretty good chance of not being affected by them, and that's probably going to see you through. So why not operate on that assumption? If you're going to ask for intervention, sometimes you can involve your life in such a concatenation of events that you're going to find misery. In my father's case, by following reasonable medical advice, he lost most of what he would have had left to him."

"How long ago was that?"

"Fifteen years."

"Did they do a CAT scan to see if it had spread?"

"I think they did some workup, but this cancer was so invidious that it had already metastasized to the brain, and it also shortly thereafter appeared to be multifocal. What was known at the time was that if you develop lung cancer, you have a less than 10 percent chance of surviving, even with early detection. So why do we *get* routine chest X rays?" He laughed. "Why do we *do* it? We do it because it's what we're trained to do. And we're trained to try to tell people what they have, as if knowledge is in itself the power of healing. Well, it isn't."

"In many instances it isn't."

"Yes, and in a few it is. I don't want to seem kooky. I *do* do things. I do have a family history of glaucoma, so I check that regularly. In other words, I will make a reasonable effort. And, if I were asked, I would urge other people to do the same in areas where they seem vulnerable and where there is reasonable medical help. In this specific thing, the possibility of prostate cancer, I'm a little uneasy about doing some kind of laboratory test that is still relatively new and that may involve me with a lot of other laboratory tests and become more trouble to me than it is worth."

"Do you get a DRE annually?"

"No. I haven't gotten annual physicals recently."

"Why not?"

"Because I think there's not much likelihood of a doctor finding anything, certainly in a young person in our society. Now, say, if tuberculosis becomes resurgent, that would be important to check out. Roughly, in the time that I was growing up, there wasn't much one would expect to find. Most people feel better to receive this card which is a sort of contract, a summary of everything our society can give people to assure them they have these grades and ratings."

"Yours is certainly an unconventional and refreshing point of view."

"I'm going to be attacked despite my pseudonymity," he said, laughing.

FEBRUARY 25, 1994. I got a call the other day from a man named Dick Murphy, who identified himself as a good friend of a friend of mine and who said he was calling at my friend's suggestion because he had recently been diagnosed with prostate cancer, and my friend had told him I might be able to offer some advice on what to do. I learned that Murphy is fifty-three; that his PSA is a little under 6; that his bone and CAT scans were negative; and that he had never heard of a Gleason score.

"Given your relatively young age," I said, "if I were in your shoes I wouldn't go for radiation. You're too young for it. The cancer may recur, and you can never repeat the radiation. Also, surgery after radiation can be complicated. I'd have a radical prostatectomy, and I'd try hard to have Patrick Walsh at Johns Hopkins do it. He has an unusually high success rate in avoiding incontinence and impotence in his patients. Also, because of your age I wouldn't delay."

"That sounds like good advice," said Dick Murphy. "In addition to yourself, I've had some people recommend Walsh. I'm going to call Johns Hopkins."

We chatted a while. He was unusually articulate, with a striking grasp of details both technical and psychological. But what especially caught my attention was that he had had three negative biopsies prior to the biopsy that had led to the diagnosis. As a consequence, I interviewed him recently in his home in a village near Princeton.

After introducing me to his blonde wife, Nora, born in Switzerland, and leaving her in the living room, he led me to the family room, with its tan leather sofa and armchairs, red brick wall and elegant bookshelves. He's tall, with a good figure and carefully barbered, silvering hair. He wore a shirt with broad maroon stripes, a maroon full-sleeve sweater, black trousers and black loafers. He spoke rapidly in a tenor voice.

"What do you do?" I asked.

"I'm an engineer."

"Aside from the cancer, is your health good?"

"Yes. Generally excellent."

"Did your father or a brother have prostate cancer?"

"My father died of prostate cancer when he was eighty-five."

"Do you remember what his Gleason score was?"

"No. My father was an Old World fellow. I was fortunate to be told he was *ill*."

"Were you having annual physicals, with a digital rectal exam?"

I probably hadn't had a physical for a year and a half or two. I was busy, and I was going with the statistics. My family was very, very healthy. All the males died of old age. On my father's side—one of my father's sisters died when she was in her sixties, I assume from cancer. This is now probably thirty-five years ago. At that time, in my family, nobody told you when people were ill, nobody told you what people died of. What I did discover since then is that first cousins of mine—it was this family of thirteen, an Irish family, a farming family, ten boys and three girls, and the three girls died of breast cancer before they reached the age of thirty-five. This was in Ireland, and we're talking about Irish Catholics. I'm part of the Murphys that emigrated to America, and they're part of the Murphys which stayed in Ireland. It was very unusual. No problem with the males.

"Can you tell me the history of your negative biopsies?"

It was probably in March of '92. I woke up. High fever. Unable to urinate. It dribbled. My wife essentially had to walk me to the toilet. I was so ill. As if I had a very bad flu. I saw the doctor within twenty-four hours. Initial diagnosis: most likely a urinary type of infection. I was treated with a sulfa drug. Within five days I was essentially almost feeling normal, with the exception of the fact that I felt a slight sensation of puffiness inside my colon area; in my rectal area.

I went back to my physician, who gave me a digital exam. He said everything felt fine. "Let's treat you a little while longer with the sulfa drug." I believe I was back again within a week or so, saying, "I'm not convinced that's my problem. I still have this sensation. I feel normal,

I have no urinary problems, I have no fever, but when I sit I feel as if I have a small whiffleball about a few inches inside my colon area."

Another doctor in the same office gave me a digital exam and said, "It feels fine. Soft, smooth." So I decided to wait another few weeks. But still the same puffiness. I decided to see a local urologist. Digital exam.

He says to me, "Did anybody check your prostate with a digital?"

I said, "Yes, I had two digitals in the last three months."

He says, "I feel some bumpiness in here. I think we should do a biopsy."

The PSA was normal—2.9, something like that. We did a biopsy. I think there were at least six, possibly eight, tissue samples taken the first time. All came back negative.

He said, "Well, there is a possibility that you could have a deep prostate infection, which is sometimes difficult to resolve."

He decided to treat me with an antibiotic, Floxin. So I did some reading on Floxin. Yes, Floxin is to be used for prostate infections over a six-week period. That's the general stretch.

The same problem existed after about six weeks. So we're probably now into late July or early August. We talked about it again, and he said, "Well, there is a possibility that it could have been bad tissue sampling. Something could have happened during the testing for the cancer cells. It's probably worthwhile to do a biopsy again." So we had another biopsy, and all the tissue samples came out negative, along with the PSA being normal.

Joining us, Nora sat down on Dick's left.

But he did say there were still these small nodules which felt a little rough. And he supposedly had tested through some of them. We then went on probably for another six to eight weeks. When he began to talk about—you know, it could be a capillary blood problem—I got the feeling he had reached the limit of his knowledge about what my problem was. So I decided to see somebody else.

I gave the new man the entire story. Two biopsies, two normals, and the particular sensation that I had, a slight puffiness—not all the time, but every now and then. He did a digital, took a semen sample, and I felt that maybe I have somebody here who indeed is going to

pursue my problem. But when I went into his office for a consulta-
tion I saw he had several folders *on his desk, and I said to myself,*
"The man is too busy." I was going on a business trip to California.
I said, "I'll return in a week." He told me that by the time I returned
he would talk with the pathologist and the first urologist, and also
would see if he could put a few things together.

When I returned, I called up, and he hadn't gotten a chance to do
it yet. I waited a few more days, and he hadn't gotten a chance to do it
again. (I was speaking to the nurse.) This went on for two and a half
more weeks, and I saw there was no result whatsoever. So I decided,
"I'd better go someplace else. I have already lost an additional month of
trying to diagnose what my problem is." Wrote him a nasty note.
Hand-delivered it. Said, "You did half the work. You get half the pay."

Dick Murphy laughed.

Then I talked to someone else locally, just as to what I'd do, and I
decided to go to Sloan-Kettering in New York. I thought it was a good
place to go. They specialize in cancer. It's a recognized institution. This
would be October of '92. Called Sloan-Kettering, talked to the urology
department, made an appointment to see somebody, was told to bring
the tissue samples from the second biopsy. They tested the samples and
they were all negative.

The doctor said, "All surgeons like to take their own tissue samples.
We'll do it again."

So I had a third biopsy, the first at Sloan-Kettering. All tissue sam-
ples were again normal, and the PSA was also within the normal
range—3.6, 3.7, something like that. I also left a semen sample, taken
by a massage of the prostate gland.

No indication of any cancer whatsoever.

He said, "Let's treat you with Floxin again. You may have a
chronic infection."

So we treated that. I went back to him six weeks later. Things felt
normal. I felt pretty good. He said, "Come back in six months." I
thought coming back in six months was reasonable. I had done a little
bit of homework, I had gone to the library to read. Six months was a rea-
sonable period of time.

247

So I went to see him. This was now in March of '93. He gave me a digital exam and said, "The gland is small, smooth and soft. PSA was normal. Come back in a year." The sensation of puffiness had gone away. Next visit was to have been in March of '94.

I spent a good summer. Things looked reasonably good. But by roughly September of '93 it began to bother me again, but this time in a slightly different fashion. I sit at a computer terminal probably a good four or five hours every day. I noticed that about three o'clock I felt some uncomfortable sensation in sitting. It was usually fine after a weekend, when I was standing, or not in a constant sitting mode. I also noticed that if there were a long weekend, generally by Wednesday it probably began to bother me. By Thursday and Friday I was uncomfortable. I was always able to alleviate the problem by standing up for a while. I decided to go back to the doctor.

I had a digital exam at Sloan-Kettering by a young urologist. He said it felt fine. Said, "Inasmuch as you've had chronic problems, let's treat you with Floxin." Gave me a prescription for a long period of time. My gut feeling was, "This is not the problem. I don't have an infection. I have something else wrong." I made an appointment to come back in December.

Went back in December, didn't see my original urologist. I saw another fellow, also a urologist. He gave me a digital exam, and he said at the time, "It feels fine." I mentioned the fact that I was taking Floxin. He told me to stop taking the Floxin, and I remember questioning him. "I was here a month ago, and somebody gave me a prescription for Floxin for three months. It's roughly five dollars a pill, and you're telling me now four weeks later to stop." So he had me take blood for my PSA number, and I said, "What am I going to do now?"

I guess it was probably two weeks after that when I got the call from the hospital. I was told my PSA was now outside of the normal range. It was now, I think, 4.9. And it was now time to take a fourth biopsy— the second at Sloan. So we drove to New York December 31. I will not forget the trip. It was just beginning the famous ice storm.

Met the doctor. After a digital he said, "There's a hard surface in here. As hard as a nut. That's where I'm going to do my biopsy."

Took his tissue samples. Also did a PSA. And I received a call, probably in the early part of January, where they told me that cancer was detected in my prostate.

I made an appointment to see the surgeon. We went to New York.

I asked, "Why did it take so long? Why did it not show up until the fourth biopsy?" I didn't get a satisfactory answer to myself.

He recommended, because of my early age, a radical prostatectomy. I actually had a very cold feeling. I just did not feel comfortable with the results that I had with my discussion. On the way home I mentioned it to my wife. What did she think? She had the same sensation herself. We agreed the doctor appeared somewhat distant.

I called Johns Hopkins, tried to make an appointment with Dr. Walsh. It was one of those things where I would have to wait four, five, or six weeks to see him. So I made an appointment with a member of his staff. I felt comfortable with this fellow.

One of the questions I asked was, "How many of these have you done?"

He said, "I do four radicals a week, and I've been doing that since 1988 or '89."

My mind quickly added it up, and I said, "That's a thousand. It sounds pretty good."

"What was your Gleason score?" I asked.

Before I spoke to you, I had never heard of a Gleason. It's 7 to 8, but not of all the tissues. Of the six tissue samples, three were positive and three were negative. Things were racing through my mind so quickly, and I was beginning to understand the seriousness of the problem. Now that it was diagnosed, I was beginning to think about, What was I going to do? I had already had an opinion; I should have a radical prostatectomy. Should I have it there? Should I wait a long time to see Patrick Walsh?

I said, "I've heard of people who do have radiation. What are the problems with that?"

He said, "Many surgeons, particularly here, will not remove a prostate after radiation therapy, because of scar tissue." So I decided we'll do a radical.

Both at Sloan and at Hopkins the decision is really because of my young age. If it's young—and I am fifty-three—the object is to remove the cancer in its entirety if possible.

He said, "The only way we're going to do that is by surgery. The radical is probably the best way to stretch out your longevity. There's no reason you cannot live a normal life cycle."

So—after, what was slightly amusing, we sat down, my wife comes in, and he starts to tell me roughly what he was going to do. And while he's telling me, I realize that all the blues, and the yellows, and greens are all beginning to turn a slight shade of gray. So I said, "I need a glass of water very quick." And I bent my head down.

He said, "No, you don't need any water. We'll get you some juice and crackers." So I had the juice, and I began to turn normal, and I apologized, and he said, "It happens to everybody."

I talked to him about retaining my libido. I said, "I understand the probabilities here are generally very good."

And with a little smile he said, "What do you want? Do you want an erection? Or do you want the cancer out?"

He said it in a way which was not harsh. What would you like? Would you like to continue sex? Or would you like to have the cancer removed? And I just chuckled to him, and I said, "Fine."

So, continuing along the same line, he said, "There are over a million men who have this problem, and there are things that you can do."

So, leading a sheltered life, I said, "What do you do?"

So he said, "You can give yourself a local injection."

And I said, "Where? In your penis?"

He said, "Yeah."

I said, "My God! I can't go to the dentist! How am I going to do that?"

My mind was spinning from giving yourself an injection in your groin area.

He said his concern is that my cancer could be erratic. It has this unusual Gleason. It could have moved to other areas around or outside the general area of the prostate.

My wife and I both feel comfortable with the surgeon. Which was different from the feeling we had when we were in New York.

I asked him about the local. I said to him, "What is the difference between a local and a general?" He said he didn't think there was too much of a problem, that what they do at Johns Hopkins is primarily a local.

He said, "If you want a general it can be done."

I said, "No. I believe it's better to be on your own breathing than to breathe through an apparatus." I said, "I'm a very sensitive and nervous person. If I know what you're doing, I'm going to get up and walk away, no matter what you're doing."

So he said, "No, you won't."

He said surgery would be between four and five hours. I remember him telling me the survival rate is 99 percent, because there's always the possibility of a problem with surgery. He said incontinency is between 3 and 5 percent. And so on.

I asked, "What caused you to pursue your problem despite the negative biopsies?"

I have an engineering background. The body is a machine. Something is not working right. And there is a reason for everything. I'm not a psychosomatic. There was a physical problem. Therefore something is wrong. I see doctors as technicians. Technicians of the body, like others are technicians of electronics, or who repair refrigerators or TVs. They just handle flesh. And I was looking to find somebody who would be able to take the sensation, or at least the criteria or data that I was telling him, and put it together with something that he may have seen before, and may give him a clue.

I would ask myself, "Why, if people are telling me my prostate is normal, why do I have the sensation at the end of the day where I feel this puffiness?" I never got an answer.

I'll step back once again. About three years ago I had a urinary problem, when I was urinating every fifteen minutes. My father died in '91. I think it was coincidental that my father was passing away. And I had constant urination and I was traveling back and forth to various hospitals. I'm generally a nervous person, and it was after I went to the urologist and looking into my bladder that he had thought at the time it was probably due to nerves, because nothing showed up any place. And then I was fine from '91 for another eighteen months or so. Whether this problem was coincidental or not, there is always a possibility, but I don't really think so, there were so many things going on in my life with my father being ill. I am a nervous individual in that area.

"Has anyone come up with a theory as to how three of your biopsies were negative?"

No. None of my urologists has been able to answer that question.

"Did you have any trouble accepting the diagnosis when it was made?"

No. It was a problem. I said to myself, "They finally found something wrong. The problem has now been identified. Let's march forward and get it corrected." The problem that I had, this feeling of puffiness, was also cyclic. It may go away for many many weeks at a time. And I may get a bad period, let's say for a week or two, where I'm very uncomfortable in the evening. And right now, I was thinking a few days ago that I have no sensation whatsoever of any problem. None. Zero.

Well, things do go through your mind when you're first diagnosed. Have I two weeks left? Ten weeks? Four? That was it. Certainly Nora, my wife, is taking it hard. And I think it really comes down to being left alone, because Nora is an only child, and I think that's part of the problem. And at night if you're awake, yourself, and you can hear your partner—I can hear my wife at times, crying.

Dick glanced rapidly at Nora, and then I did. Her face was contorted with silent weeping. She covered her face with her hands, and after a moment left the room.

That was the most difficult part. Not the fact that I have cancer, which I believe I've dealt with, and can deal with, but those individuals who are left behind, particularly my wife. That is the only remorse or regret that I have. My current PSA is 5.7. Very, very gradual, this rise. Since I cannot go back, I cannot undo anything. I made a decision. I feel comfortable. And we'll go with the decision, we'll go with the results.

"Do you have any advice to offer to someone who's freshly diagnosed with cancer?"

If you think you have a problem, pursue it. Do not give up. Do not listen to your urologist. Your body tells you there's something wrong. Pursue it, if you have to pursue it with a second doctor, or a third doctor. If you have cancer, it's not the end of the world. Make your decision. But always go for a second opinion. And listen to other individuals who have prostate cancer, and find out what they have had done. I've spoken with many people about my problem. I've told my story, oh, a dozen times. I think it's somewhat of a mission to tell other individuals that you should be pursuing the problem. You should be getting your PSA every year when you go for a physical. If you think you have a problem, pursue it. Don't be fooled because you don't have any pain.

Most of the people I've talked to, whom I've known for years, have told me that with the three biopsies, they wouldn't have pursued it. They would have gone with the conclusion that you've got chronic prostatitis. I just like to be aggressive. I felt it was a medical problem. Doctors are just like people. They go home and have cocktails, they have kids, they have good days and bad. So if you go to this guy, it could have been his bad day. Pursue it.

I think I'm dealing with my problem well, and I don't know why. But I might attribute part of it to an individual by the name of Wally Starlock, a bright head, an intellect, someone I've worked with for a number of years. We've talked about life, death, religion, the herelife, the afterlife, what we should do, what we should not do.

It turns out that the philosophy is that you're here for a particular period of time. If it's eighty years, great. If it's fifty years, great. Maybe there isn't anything to miss in between. Those of us who are here after us will continue to pursue it. And in many cases you may do better when you're gone than when you're here.

Nora reappeared. Her face showed no sign of tears. "You're doing fine," Dick said to her softly. Turning back to me, he continued his story.

I'll just take whatever period of time there is, and enjoy it. It's diagnosed, it's over, I'll just have to pursue it. And let's go with it. Certainly there was great remorse. Not the question of why me? But the question of, why wasn't it discovered earlier, when I had seen whom I believe to be qualified physicians?

After three or four weeks, this dark cloud passed. What helped, and I told this to someone else at work who was recently diagnosed with bone cancer, is talking to everybody. I talked to all my friends at work. And it was good. People came up to me and said, "I hear you have a problem." I would just tell them what the problem is, and go through the entire story as I did with you. And talking about it helps. Don't keep it a secret. It helps to talk to people. I tell everybody. I tell the whole thing about the rising penis, where the needle goes. [Laughter.] I just talk.

One other thing I've also noticed. I generally had a good Catholic upbringing. When you've been told you have cancer, it brings back a real sense of mortality. That eventually you'll have to finally meet your Maker. And that if you believe in a hereafter, you'll have to be judged. It's something to think about very hard, particularly if you do know there's an illness that may terminate your life early.

So . . . in my particular case . . . I think I've made peace with God. . . . And I think I've made peace . . . with everybody.

Dick walked me to my car. It had been a fine interview. But it had been more than that. I had come to like him a lot, and to empathize strongly with his and his wife's fears.

Fifteen

March 4 to August 8, 1994

MARCH 4, 1994. I had blood drawn this morning for a PSA test and an acid phosphatase. (Today is exactly nine months since I finished radiation therapy.) Suspense. Will my new PSA be low? High? I feel caught by the PSA flypaper. What if my PSA climbs? Will it mean watchful waiting, with the probability, somewhere down the road, of hormonal therapy? I suppose so.

When I spoke with a friend of mine recently, I asked how her husband is. He's the man who had cryosurgery a year ago. "He's fine," she said. After a pause she added, "He's impotent. Permanently. He's made his peace with it." I gather she's made her peace with it too.

MARCH 10, 5:00 P.M. I still haven't heard from Dr. North about my latest PSA. He usually calls promptly. Is he very busy? Or does his silence mean the number has risen, and he prefers to give it to me in person?

5:45 P.M. I called his house and spoke with his wife, who paged him on a beeper. Calling within a quarter of an hour, he explained he had been very busy.

"Your new PSA is 4.4," he said. "I'm very pleased, because essentially this is equivalent to your last one, 4.0. PSA can easily

255

vary. A particularly hard stool on the morning you had blood drawn could account for the 4.4. Next time it may be 3.8. If it had suddenly gone to 7 or 8, I would want to find out why. What matters is where your PSA levels off for your particular baseline."

I was greatly relieved. I told myself not to worry about my PSA from now on; that the radiation had worked; and was probably still working; and would continue to do so for at least a year after therapy.

MARCH 14, 1994. I met with him this morning. "What's my acid phosphatase?" I asked.

"2.8."

"It's gone up a bit. Last time it was 2.3."

"It fluctuates, like PSA. Like blood pressure. Very little significance, if any, in so little a change."

"What's the normal range?"

"1.8 to 3.8. Any urinary discomfort?"

"No."

"Frequency?"

"Good."

"At night?"

"Much better than before radiation."

"Stream?"

"Better."

"Erection?"

"Normal."

"Good!"

"What's the percentage of radiation-caused impotence? 25 to 50?"

"Fifty is too high a figure. A recent study put it at 28."

"What do you predict for my next PSA?"

"Your PSA may be bottoming out. At 4 . . . 4.5 . . . 5 . . . It may fluctuate by plus or minus one point."

That was very good news. I felt high when I left him.

MARCH 23, 1994. Today was my first visit to the King City prostate cancer support group since the end of June, nine months ago. Some twenty people were present, including five spouses. This is the largest attendance I have seen at this group. Many of the people were new to me.

The chief item on today's agenda was a talk about Eulexin (flutamide) by a representative of the drug's manufacturer, who explained that Eulexin blocks the androgen (sex hormone) produced by the adrenal glands from attaching itself to receptors in the prostate, thus helping to starve prostatic cancer. He said Eulexin is designed to be used only in conjunction with Lupron or a similar testosterone-suppressing drug. The representative was a large, full-bellied, brown-skinned man who looked to be of Hindu origin. He spoke without an accent.

"Can't you pharmaceutical people help us women deal with our irritable spouses?" Dolly Lombardi interrupted in an aggressive tone, frowning heavily. "The hormone treatment has changed them."

She's Henry Lombardi's wife. I had met her briefly when I interviewed him early in January. Her tone and demeanor surprised me. The rep too was surprised. He raised his brows, shaking his head negatively, slowly.

"I wish we could help. . . ." he said lamely. "I don't know of anything that's being done in that line. . . ."

"Well, put your minds to it!" said Dolly almost hostilely, again surprising me.

Why haven't I sensed earlier that she's a strong lady? And why was she sitting so far apart from Henry? Henry, smiling gently in his fashion, and wearing his full head of pure-white hair, looked content as he leaned forward the better to hear any further exchanges.

A man on a sofa opposite mine (his face was in silhouette because of the intense outdoor light behind him) said, "Either physical castration—or medical castration—changes us. No libido. No need or desire to fondle. I don't think anything can be done about it. That's it!"

"It's pitiful," remarked a woman bitterly who was sitting in the middle of the large room. Gray-haired, she wore an off-white dress. Her spouse, sitting beside her, wore a suit and tie. Studying his lap, he seemed to be hanging his head in embarrassment.

"The medical profession should address itself to this problem," said a man. "Perhaps a calming medication can be given together with the Lupron and Eulexin, or after an orchiectomy."

"I'm almost eighty-six, and I don't think pills are the answer," disagreed the gentleman on my left who was sharing the sofa with me. "The couples need to work on their minds and emotions."

Surprisingly, the rep launched into an attack on President Clinton's health plan, getting increasingly heated. He said that, as a result of living in England for several years, he had concluded that the English health care system is not only a medical failure but is bankrupting the nation. His remarks were greeted with polite silence.

MARCH 31. Last evening, at around midnight, I strained myself carrying a female classmate's heavy portfolio and heavy camera bags and placing them on the back seat of her car, leaning over to do so. Something seemed to give in my groin, and I tried to pay no attention to it, but within the hour I was shocked by the sight of bright blood in my urine, which took a while to stop. I had never experienced a flow of blood in my urine. I felt shaky, cold. The blood didn't recur during the night. I'm drinking lots of herb tea to flush my urinary system, and am watching my urine closely. So far, no further signs of trouble.

APRIL 14, 1994. Early in April Cousin Erik called to advise me not to rush into telling Dr. North about the blood in my urine.

"There's no way he can reassure you without a test," said Erik. "And you may not want to get involved in a cystoscopy yet."

For a couple of days there was no spotting, but then I was upset to discover traces in my underpants. And there were continuing traces during the next several days. So I called Dr. North today, explained, and at his advice left a urine specimen at the hospital for a urinalysis.

What can the blood mean? Where is it coming from? My bladder? My prostate? My urethra? My penis? Can it be due to the little accident I had when lifting the portfolio and camera bags onto the back seat? Or to my often squatting at the Cibachrome class because I keep my safe box on the floor when I'm at my enlarger station? (I mentioned these speculations to Dr. North.) Can the blood be related to my prostate cancer? To the radiation? It's weird to see my body behaving so strangely, and to have no firm inkling as to the cause.

APRIL 15, MORNING. Phoning nurse Debby Kuban, who looked up the results on the computer for me, I learned that my urinalysis and urine culture were both normal. A relief! I'll call Dr. North this afternoon to see what this means. Later. Joan said he called, and wants me to continue my "lifestyle," and that he suspects that the strain I had on lifting the portfolio and camera bags, or the squatting at the Cibachrome class, *may* have caused my urine-blood symptoms.

During the first ten days of May I almost felt I was being teased by the spotting, which occurred . . . then disappeared . . . then occurred . . . then disappeared . . . in a seemingly chaotic fashion.

On May 9, in preparation for my annual physical with Dr. Redmont (my internist, or all-around medical caretaker), I had blood drawn at the hospital for my PSA and acid phosphatase. On May 12, while I was in Dr. Redmont's office for the exam, a female nurse called the hospital, got my latest PSA reading, and gave it to him.

It was 11.5!

"I'm shocked!" I said to him. "On March 4 it was 4.4."

"There's nothing to be upset about," said Dr. Redmont calmly.

The remark was uncharacteristic of him; he's usually a worrier.

When he suggested we repeat the PSA, this time in *his* lab, I declined, saying I had had it done only three days ago.

I called Dr. North's home early that evening, and he phoned back and said there were five possibilities regarding my PSA's rise.

(1) The latest PSA was an error.

(2) It was an example of PSA's ability to fluctuate dramatically.

(3) My PSA was returning to my BPH (benign prostatic hypertrophy; benign enlargement of the gland) baseline; which was to say, 4.0 and 4.4 were "eccentric."

"We know your gland is very large," he said. "Maybe the benign cells of your prostate were injured by the radiation to the extent where they stopped producing PSA. And now they're recovering and producing it."

(4) The radiation had failed.

(5) The worst-case scenario: the cancer may have gone into bone.

"But even if that happened, we can use hormone suppressors," he said. "They cause side effects, but can give you five or ten more years of life. We don't know enough yet about PSA to predict its behavior well. I don't believe your latest PSA indicates cancer. Also, an isolated PSA reading is not very meaningful. What's necessary is to discover a trend by the use of several PSA readings over a period of months. When the new reading came across my desk, I called Lew Gilroy about it, and we concluded that on your return from California in July, you'll have a PSA test in his office, on his new machine. If the PSA is high, he'll do an ultrasound and figure out your PSA density, which is the PSA over the gland's volume. My advice is, try to relax. "

I tried to relax, but it wasn't easy to keep from wondering if my radiation therapy had failed, and if I had made a mistake in not going for a prostatectomy. But in a while, calming down, I returned to my belief that at my age a prostatectomy would have been the wrong choice.

"Maybe, considering my age, I should have chosen watchful waiting," I thought.

But a problem for me was that, except on arising from a night's sleep, when I felt stiff and achy, I didn't *feel* my chronological age, so it was often difficult to remember to *think* it, to think, "You're an old man, closing in on the end, so there's little if any point in getting worked up about a rise in your PSA."

MAY 16, 1994. Meeting with Dr. North this morning, I asked, "What's my latest acid phosphatase reading?"

"Oddly enough, it went down: 2.2."

"What does that mean?"

Smiling, he rotated his index finger at the side of his head.

"Is it possible there's a connection between the rise in my PSA and the recent traces of blood in my urine?"

"Yes. If you had a mild prostatitis, it would increase your PSA and might produce the blood. As for the traces of blood, I think it was probably very minor. Remember, when we recently did a urinalysis, there were no red cells. And your even more recent urinalysis with Daniel Redmont was also negative. The neck of your bladder got quite a beating by the radiation, so it wouldn't surprise me if the mucosa got thinned a bit, and leak a little occasionally. Keep a watch. If there's a change, if there's a considerable amount of blood, then you'll need a cystoscopy."

"I want to avoid a cystoscopy if it's at all possible. It's an invasive procedure, and I'm sure it will result in cystitis or prostatitis or both."

"I understand."

"Is it possible the traces of blood were due to my sucking breath sweeteners; that the sweeteners contain something that acts like an antihistamine? We know that an antihistamine is contraindicated for an enlarged prostate. I once used one, Seldane, that brought blood in my urine, and when I stopped using it, the blood also stopped."

"You know the old story about the horse's hooves?"

"No."

"You're at home and you hear hooves outside. You imagine the sound is made by a horse, not a zebra, because where you live, a zebra is very uncommon. It's the same thing in medicine. What you look for first is the obvious. I learned about zebra while I was in medical school, where we used to call a far-out theory a zebra theory. In short, the connection between the traces of blood in your urine and your use of breath sweeteners is, in my opinion, a zebra."

I laughed. I felt greatly reassured by what he had said.

I had assumed that this was my last follow-up meeting with him. After all, almost a year had passed since the completion of my therapy. I felt lucky to have gotten to know him, not only because he was an excellent physician but also because he was a splendid human being. After our exchange about blood, PSA and acid phosphatase, we had a pleasant chat about nonmedical matters, during which I was relieved to learn we would continue to meet regularly for another year.

MAY 24, 1994. The prostate cancer support group convened this afternoon at the Franklin House as usual. Fourteen people attended, five of them women. Dr. North gave a lecture on the use of strontium 89 for pain in bone metastases not only from prostate cancer but from other cancers as well. It was a pleasure for me to introduce him.

Generally, pain from bone metastases develops over a period of weeks and months. Usually, at first, it's treated with nonsteroidal anti-

inflammatories like Motrin and Tylenol. It starts intermittently; it's unrelated to activity; and, interestingly, it's more severe at night. It becomes progressively severe. It's usually localized; a patient will have, on a bone scan, a particular area that's hot. He may have a pain that he can point to, and when the physician percusses the area, it's tender. When the disease gets more advanced, and there are more hot spots, sometimes people don't describe, "Well, this hurts me, and this hurts me." They say, "I hurt all over."

Occasionally we hear, "One day my shoulder hurts so bad. Then the next day that pain is gone, and I have a pain in my leg." That's a migratory-pain syndrome. And what I feel is happening in that case is that the patient's brain is able to focus on only one or two pain sites at any one time. If you burn your hand while cooking, and it's excruciatingly painful, and then you stub your toe, all of a sudden you forget about the pain in your hand, because your toe is hurting.

Sometimes it's a generalized, I-can't-vocalize-it type of pain. That, actually, is the hardest type of pain for a radiation oncologist to treat, because as we aim our beam here on one day, we think we're doing great work, because the next day, after one treatment, that pain is gone. But it's replaced by another pain, and so we're doing some tail-chasing. That is just the ideal situation for using strontium 89.

Usually bone scans show areas of increased activity. Bone scans are very sensitive; but they're not all that specific; arthritis may look just like a bone metastasis. It depends on where the sites are; on the number; and on how they change over time. Bone scans can look wildly positive; whereas the X rays can look quite clear. CAT scans sometimes help us determine bone metastasis. And sometimes it will be bone scan activity, together with a rise in PSA, that will diagnose metastatic prostate cancer.

Bone pain is a nonspecific finding. Everybody gets some bone pain. So, if a man has prostate cancer and now has a pain in the hip, it's nonspecific. It's more likely to be arthritis or muscle pain. We don't use just clinical symptoms as a diagnostic.

What are the therapeutic options for metastatic prostate cancer and the pain it generates? Nonsteroidals, like Motrin, are effective for minimal to mild pain. Left without treatment, the pain continues, gradually becomes more and more intermittent, and then becomes more severe. Chemotherapy is not an overwhelmingly wonderful option for prostate cancer. There are some drugs that do help, but their toxicity profile can be excessive, and it's awfully hard to justify putting a man through the toxicity of chemotherapy for a 20 percent response rate. Generally, hormonal manipulation is excellent, but the median duration of hormonal manipulation suppressing prostate cancer is about two years, after which the cancer cells will start to outgrow the suppression. They will become what we call hormone-resistant.

Analgesics and narcotics are the mainstay of treating bone pain for metastases. The obvious downsides of narcotics are, they impair people's lifestyles. They make you constipated, and that's the most common and most debilitating side effect of narcotics. Nerve blocks are a newer modality. We can inject nerves that are being invaded, or are being compressed by bone disease. Nerve blocks actually kill the nerves. So it's a way of stopping our perception of pain. The same thing happens with narcotics. Narcotics dull our sensation of pain.

Local radiotherapy is an important means for treating metastatic prostate cancer. It's very easy to do, and it's generally easy for the patient to tolerate. It's often given in ten treatments. The response rates are about 80 to 90 percent. So, for men who have pain from metastatic prostate cancer, if we can localize it we can treat it, and there's an 80 to 90 percent chance that the treatment will achieve maximum pain relief within a matter of several weeks.

Strontium 89 is really an ideal product for what I want to talk about. It has a short half-life—about 50.5 days—in contradistinction to one of its parents, strontium 90, which, you may remember, was a radioactive fallout product of nuclear testing. Strontium 90 contaminated the surface of ground, and has a half-life of thousands of years. When cows ate the grass that had been contaminated, they produced strontium 90 in their milk, which babies then drank, and those babies, now grown adults, are radioactive.

By contrast, strontium 89 is a beautiful drug for suppressing metastatic bone pain, for one reason because it has a very short range in tissue, in the order of about 2 or 3 millimeters. So it's a way of giv-

PSA for his new PSA machine. (Heretofore I've always had the PSA done at the hospital.) This is my first PSA after the worrisome one of 11.5 on May 9. Helen, his office manager, said she'd have the result by today.

What will my new reading be? 17? 18? Maybe even 20? I won't be surprised if it is. After all, I know of at least two cases in the King City support group in which cancer recurred after radiation. However, in those it returned five or six years *after* radiation. So why am I jumping the gun?

Let's assume my latest PSA is 18. What will that mean for me? No doubt a bone scan. Maybe also a CAT scan. Also an MRI? Followed by a period of watchful waiting? For how long? And then what? Medical castration (Lupron and Eulexin)? Or surgical castration? Will I seriously entertain the latter? Why not? At my age, impotence is not far off in any event. But how will castration affect my ability to continue to work creatively?

"Give Helen a call," I tell myself. "Face the music."

But I keep stalling. I'm feeling good and am working well, so why throw myself into a paroxysm of anxiety, of decision-making, of arranging appointments for a battery of tests? I deserve a period free of all that. Deserve? Cancer doesn't give a damn about what I deserve.

Shortly before noon I make the call, thinking, "Maybe Helen is already out to lunch, and I'll have an hour or two more of respite."

But she answers.

"Helen, what's my PSA?"

"Wait just a moment. I need to go over to Diane and get the number from her. She's the one who handles it."

I wait. Helen seems to be taking a long time. Is she shocked by the number? Or was the 11.5 a clerical error, and will I drop to 5, 6, 7—numbers I expect are normal for me, with my very large gland? Increasingly anxious, I'm almost ready to hang up. At last I hear her picking up the phone.

"Mr. Neider, it's 3.39," she says in a matter-of-fact tone.

"3.39?" I repeat skeptically.

I have trouble believing her; or believing my ears.

"Yes, 3.39."

I feel like shouting, "That's wonderful! Unbelievable!" But I don't. Instead, I say quietly, "That's pretty good. Thanks a lot, Helen."

Hanging up, I think, "So Daniel Redmont was right when he said, 'It's nothing to be concerned about.' But on what basis did he say it? Did he have something in mind, or was it just a chance remark? 3.39! This is the lowest it's ever been for me! And this is the first time I've encountered a PSA with *two* decimal numbers. That 9 stands for 9 hundredths of a billionth of a gram of the antigen! What a measuring system!"

I felt I had to share my good news with somebody. Joan was at the Y, swimming, so I couldn't immediately convey the news to her. I left a message for Dr. North at the Oncology Center; called Susy, my daughter; Mark, my brother; Tessie, my sister; Cousin Erik; and crossed the street and told my friend Bernie. Everyone was surprised and pleased.

To celebrate, I bought some Nova Scotia belly lox, a sourdough boule, a six-pack of Sierra Nevada Pale Ale, and some coffee ice cream. As soon as Joan entered the house she cried, "Congratulations!" and hugged me.

"How do you know?" I asked.

"Susy was at the Y. She told me. She thought she shouldn't, that *you* should tell me, but she couldn't hold the news back. I shouldn't have told you that I know."

"No, it's fine."

"3.39! Now that's a *number!*" she cried.

What a relief! No more spotting! No more current worries about the possibility of castration or hormonal therapy!

In the evening I noticed large, deep bruises on my right arm where Dr. Gilroy had withdrawn blood. Clearly he wasn't as adept at this procedure as the nurses at the hospital.

JULY 22, FRIDAY. I decided it would be wise to have another PSA, this time at the hospital for the sake of consistency and comparison. When I called Dr. North and explained, he agreed with me, so I picked up a prescription at the Oncology Center and had blood drawn this afternoon.

JULY 26. During my visit to Dr. Gilroy today, he began with a series of questions.

"Appetite?"

"Good."

"Any pain in urinating?"

"No."

"Any dribbling?"

"No."

"Any accidents?"

"No."

"Bowel movements. Any pain?"

"No."

"Control?"

"Good."

"Accidents?"

"No."

He had me lie on a gurney while he thumped and pummeled various parts of my torso, frequently asking, "Pain here?" My reply was always "No."

He did a digital, then said, "Your prostate feels good. Good consistency. Good symmetry. And no protuberance. It's still a large gland, but the volume has been reduced by about a third. This is thirteen months since you finished radiation. Let's see . . . your most recent PSA was 3.39. That's good. I wouldn't be surprised if it goes to 3, or to 4 or 5. If it stays around 4 or 5, I'd say we have a cure. Charley, I'm happy with your prostate situation. See me in six months. I don't need to see you before then. If I thought I did, I'd say so."

JULY 28, 1994, JOAN'S BIRTHDAY. Our phone was out of order today, probably due to a recent storm, so I couldn't receive the call from Dr. North (regarding my newest PSA) that I thought he might be trying to make.

"Have I opened a Pandora's box?" I wondered. "Wouldn't it have been wise to let well enough alone and be happy with the 3.39? Maybe the 3.39 is a clerical error. Who knows what the new number may turn out to be? Now I've made myself anxious again."

Using an outside pay phone, I called nurse Debby Kuban at the Oncology Center and asked her to look up my latest PSA on the computer, and to tell Dr. North about my phone situation.

She called back to say my PSA is 2.8! This is my lowest PSA in many, many years!

However, I assume the difference between 2.8 and 3.39 is due not to a real decline in my PSA but rather to the difference between PSA machines and/or systems. Still, I'm genuinely surprised. And relieved.

And mystified, for isn't 2.8 rather low, given my age, together with the fact I have a very large gland? I must ask Ed North about this.

What did cause that unnerving spike of 11.5? The strain injury I had the night when there was fresh blood in my urine? My squatting at the Cibachrome class? The thinned mucosa in the neck of my bladder? And so on. . . . Speculations ad infinitum. . . .

AUGUST 8, 1994. Dr. North called, excited about my 2.8 PSA. I'll have my next PSA test on January 22, 1995, six months after my July one. I have six months in which to relax about my prostate cancer.

Sixteen

January 9, 1995

JANUARY 9, 1995. When I had a follow-up visit with Dr. North the morning of January 2, he did a digital, after which he pronounced my gland to be "Good! It's soft. It's normal."

"It's nineteen months since I finished therapy," I said. "I wonder what my new PSA will be. I won't be surprised if it goes back to 11.5, or even higher. It won't matter if it does. I'll be eighty the middle of this month, and at eighty there's little point in getting exercised about a PSA."

"Why are you being pessimistic?" he asked with a concerned smile. "I'm sure it'll be normal."

I had blood drawn on the 5th. He called this afternoon to say my latest PSA is 3.4, and that my acid phosphatase is 2.2.

"I'm delighted!" he said. "As far as I'm concerned, you have a cure! Given the fluctuation of PSA machines, 3.4 is as good as your last PSA, which was 2.8."

"Terrific!" I said. "You were right when you predicted my new PSA would be normal!"

"Congratulations!"

I've wondered, from time to time, how to end this story, and have concluded that it has no formal ending, for who knows what the next several years may bring if I survive them? And so I've decided that this, a high note, is as good a place to end as any. I'm one of the lucky ones. My prostate was watched early, and the cancer was diagnosed while it was still "curable," and at a relatively late stage of my long life. Time to say, "So far, so good."

But before I end the narrative, I'd like to share a recent conversation I had with Dr. North, in which I asked questions that had been on my mind for some time. We talked, as usual, in one of the little exam rooms of the King City Radiation Oncology Center.

"If, due to radiation, the gland shrinks, does this affect the volume of semen produced?" I asked.

Good question. Probably not from the prostate shrinking. But since I do treat the seminal vesicles, the volume of seminal fluid may be altered.

"Assuming the gland does shrink, what's the likely mechanism? Are sloughed-off cancer cells sent into the urethra and excreted via urine?"

Cancer cells that die are digested, chewed up, by the body's immune system. Macrophages, white blood cells, come in to destroy them. That's what causes some prostatitis, the inflammation during and shortly after the treatment. Even now, if the cell dies months after having been irradiated, the immune system will come in and chew up and remove the cells. There are some cancers that do slough off, but not that particular one.

"We talk about stages B1 and B2. B1 is for prostate cancer involving one lobe, B2 for cancer involving two lobes. We know, histologically, there are five lobes, but we never talk about the other three. Why is that?"

We can feel the two posterior ones when we do a digital. We can't feel the central or the anterior lobes.

"What about the ultrasound?"

The ultrasound can see anteriorly. It's the tumor's size that's important, and not so much a designation of number of lobes. You can have a B2 that will be in only one lobe, if the tumor is larger than 2 centimeters. The classic small nodule is defined as up to 2 centimeters.

If it gets to be more than a nodule that you can palpate, and comprises an entire lobe, we still call it a B2. When I discuss it with people, I usually say, "B1 is one lobe, B2 is two lobes," because that's usually how one feels it. If it gets much more than 2 centimeters, it almost has to extend into another lobe, unless it's just going up and down, longitudinally, in the lobe.

"With aggressive radiation therapy such as I've had, is it usual to have so dramatic a change as mine?"

More often than not, it is. There's a varying spectrum of people with prostate cancer. There's a group who have a PSA that's less than 10. There's a group like you, who have a PSA between 10 and 20. And there are people who have PSAs much higher than 20. Now, I often see PSAs that are higher drop to the same levels. So their response is even more dramatic. A PSA that starts at 7 and goes to 4 is not as dramatic a response, but nonetheless the endpoint is still that we have a normal PSA. The radiation damage to the cancer cells is there, and it's permanent. The cells will continue to live until they try to divide. Some of those cells, which may still be cancer, that were left—and if we were to biopsy them, yes, we might find cancer cells—but they are rendered nonclonogenic, they can't divide, and if they decide to go through the cell cycle a month or two months from now, they will disappear and will no longer be producing PSA. So, it's not unusual, even as long as twelve to eighteen months after the conclusion of radiation, to have cancer cells that have been lethally irradiated then go through cell division and die.

"May some radiation side effects show up later?"

Yes. Maybe side effects isn't the right term. There are acute or early radiation reactions, and there are late ones. Early radiation reactions I call side effects. The early tissue reactions occur very early on, during the treatment. I call those side effects—the burning when you urinate, the diarrhea, et cetera. The late tissue reactions occur through a different process. Instead of calling them side effects I call them complications. You can get them months or years after the treatment, and those are rectal ulcers, bladder ulcers, impotence, bowel obstruction, things like that. Generally something will bring it on. A particularly hard stool, straining, may precipitate an ulcer in the rectum. It breaks down the mucosa, and then it doesn't heal as quickly, and in the meantime an infection can set up shop. Now, those late reactions are very unusual, and they may be even more unusual when we use customized conformal blocks, when we use the CT for dosimetry and target planning. We try to minimize the dose specifically to those sensitive tissues. But nonetheless, about 1 to 3 percent of the time, we see late tissue reactions. They usually do heal with time. On very rare occasions they don't heal, and we need surgery to remove the ulceration. But to require surgery for a radiation complication is extremely unusual, because you need a rare event happening on top of a rare event.

"What drugs could I have taken to alleviate some of the side effects?"

Anusol suppositories. Proctofoam for rectal irritation. For bladder irritation we often use Advil, Pyridium, occasionally Hytrin. Hytrin is useful if the bladder isn't emptying completely, if it's just filling up so quickly because it's only getting rid of 25 percent or so of its volume. The increased urine frequency isn't because you're making more urine, it's because the bladder isn't emptying completely, so it's filling more quickly. Then there are antispasmodic medications to help relax the sphincters—things like that.

"Is it possible, by the use of drugs, to avoid all such side effects?"

I've never used the drugs prophylactically, to try to prevent side effects. I don't know if they would. They might mask certain things that we would want to know. If someone gets a side effect earlier than I would anticipate, then I'd use that as a key to make sure all the calculations were rechecked. I would use the side effects as a cross-check. That's a very gross, inaccurate side-check, but if someone started getting extreme urinary or rectal irritation the first week of treatment, I would use that to go back and relook at everything. So I'm not sure I'd want to mask things to begin with.

"What are some of the percentages of prostate cancer recurrence after radiation?"

Well, there's local recurrence, and then there's systemic recurrence; recurrence in the prostate gland, and recurrence in bones. We have data on both. But one has to factor in the Gleason score, and the initial PSA, and all that, to predict for a risk of systemic disease. And since radiation and surgery—and they're often compared—are local modalities, it's best to look at local control. The recurrence rate, let's say for ten years in the prostate gland following radiation, is dependent on the size of the lesion, the stage. For Stage B the local control is about 90 to 92 percent. So the recurrence rate in the prostate gland is about 8 percent. For Stage C it's significantly higher. It may be as high as 20, 23, 25 percent recurrence rate in the gland.

I read aloud a quote from *Men's Health* magazine of December 1993 dealing with the Mayo Clinic's findings about the normal cutoff for PSA rising with each decade; to wit, 2.5 for men in their forties; 3.5 for men in their fifties; 4.5 for men in their sixties; and 6.5 for men in their seventies.

"What do you think of it?" I asked.

That's median. That's what I was saying. People are thinking that we should move the bell-shaped curve up up up as age increases. I agree that we cannot take a man who is seventy years old and who has a PSA of 5, and say, "This is abnormally high." We have to take it in the context of the situation. Again, our knowledge of it is evolving. If a year earlier it had been 3 and it's now 5, I would work that up, because BPH doesn't nearly double in one year. But if we were getting a baseline of a seventy-year-old who's never had a PSA and it's 5.0, if I didn't feel anything on a digital exam, I think I'd repeat the PSA in six months. And if it's 5, well, yes, we aren't confined, what is normal is no longer being defined by an arbitrary cutoff of 4 to extend to all men. So I agree that we should modify what a "normal" PSA is for different age groups.

"Would there be an important advantage in getting a sonogram, and comparing the size of my prostate before and after therapy?"

It could be interesting. But is there an advantage to doing it? No. There's nothing of value therapeutically to know exactly what the size is, except for your own knowledge. I wouldn't get any value out of it in terms of making decisions about your care. I wouldn't use an ultra-sound response to tell me whether things look either good or bad.

"Do you believe there's a current prostate cancer epidemic in the United States?"

Prostate cancer is related to old age. More people are living long enough to develop prostate cancer. That's one factor. I think we do have an older population now than we did thirty, forty years ago. I think that with PSA, we're picking up lots of men who would not have had their cancers diagnosed perhaps until after they died—at time of an autopsy. And so we're identifying more men with prostate cancer because of PSA. But I don't really think that means more men are getting prostate cancer. It means that more men are having it picked up at an early stage that's curable. An epidemic means, in my mind, a rapid acceleration in the incidence. Yes, there is a higher number of patients detected with it, but I don't know that it's a higher occurrence of prostate cancer. That's not gospel, though. I'm not an epidemiologist, I haven't studied the figures that closely.

"Is there a theory about why American blacks have a very high incidence of prostate cancer, much higher than African blacks?"

I don't know the theory behind it, but it seems that their lesions tend to be more aggressive, they have higher Gleason scores. It may be related to the RAS oncogene. The RAS seems to be expressed higher among black men with prostate cancer than among white. But why that seems to be the case, I don't know.

"Do you see any connection between the joint 'epidemic' of breast and prostate cancers?"

I think that diagnosis is improving with both. Mammograms are becoming not only better technically but more widely used, so we're detecting breast cancer at an earlier stage, nonpalpable versus when it was palpable. Also, I do think there probably is an increase in the actual occurrence of breast cancer.

"Does prostate cancer differ in any significant way from other cancers?"

It probably has the slowest median doubling time of most cancers. By median I mean, someone's prostate cancer may divide faster than another person's other kind of cancer; but overall, prostate cancer seems to be the most slow-growing. By the way, the earlier one's age, the more aggressively prostate cancer tends to behave.

"What changes in understanding and therapy do you foresee for prostate cancer within the next decade?"

There's so much happening at the molecular level these days, with understanding of the genetics, chromosomal mapping, banding techniques to identify genes that make one at risk for developing prostate cancer, or any kind of cancer. Every week there's a new disease that's being located in the genes. I think that a lot of our understanding is going to change about cancer in general as our understanding on the molecular level improves. How will that translate into therapy? It's going to take years, probably, but ultimately our treatment of cancer will be prevention.

"What about radiation therapy in the next decade?"

It's a very quickly evolving field. Radiation therapy today is a lot different than it was five or ten years ago. I don't anticipate a major change in the hardware technology. We'll get a little bit of higher energy here and there. Machines may get a bit smaller. I think progress will be made in using computers to target more precisely; using conformal blocks, perhaps, with computer control of the blocks; having blocks change as the machine moves around the body. And perhaps we'll see the integration of radiation implants with external beams for more advanced disease.

"Does prostate cancer kill by invading vital organs?"

That's a very good question. When it spreads, it can invade vital organs and cause those organs to shut down. When it invades the bones, people have pain, and if the pain isn't well controlled they take pain medication, and pain medication can . . . there's a whole mechanism. People tend to be more susceptible to infections, to pneumonias, to other things like that which can overcome their bodies more easily. And their nutrition isn't as good when they have pain. They're in a catabolic state. They don't mount an immune response as well, because they're not taking as much protein because of pain, and their appetite's gone. It's a difficult process to describe exactly what kills someone. We don't know—unless it has invaded a vital organ, like the brain or the lungs or the liver. But that's very late in the disease. That's why many men don't die of prostate cancer but with it, because even when it spreads, you can percolate on for many, many years without it invading a vital organ. But generally, when it gets to a certain point, the patient's performance seems to deteriorate, and he seems to be prone to infections that you and I wouldn't find overwhelming.

"What cancers do you treat other than prostate cancer?"

Everything. I'll take you from head to toe. Brain tumors. Brain metastases. Lots of head and neck cancers. Cancer of the tongue. Cancer of the larynx. Lung cancer. Esophageal cancer. Breast cancer. Colorectal cancer. Testicular cancer. Just about every malignancy into which radiation can be incorporated either definitively, adjuvantly or palliatively.

"What are your greatest rewards in your oncological work?"

A good question. The charge I get out of work is making a connection with patients no matter where they are in terms of their understanding of the cancer or their acceptance of it; helping to educate them, and knowing that I've helped them through a difficult period in their life. I know when I've made that connection, and that's what I find rewarding. Of course, I get a charge out of seeing PSAs normalize. That's a real boost to my emotional well-being. It's the sense of helping people through difficult times, whether it's through cure or through palliation; relieving the awful symptoms that are deteriorating the quality of life. That's the reward. That's the charge.

"Do you have an opinion regarding the possible relationship between antioxidants and prostate cancer?"

I don't know of any correlation, but if people told me ten years from now that ingesting lots of vitamin C seemed to lower the prostate cancer, I'd believe it, it makes some sense. However, it's only speculation.

"And now my last question. If we don't know what causes prostate cancer, how can you be sure mine won't return, even though I may be cancer-free now?"

We can't be sure. There is no guarantee. You're left with your prostate gland with the same competing forces that caused it to become malignant in the first place. The same causes may cause it to become malignant again. We don't know. All we can do is say that statistically we know that men who have good responses to PSA, to digital rectal exam, et cetera, et cetera, generally don't develop a recurrence. But if you lived another seventy years you'd probably develop another prostate cancer.

Glossary

acid phosphatase: short for prostatic acid phosphatase or serum acid phosphatase; normal range is 1.8 to 3.8. An enzyme detected in the serum produced by prostate cells.

adenocarcinoma: an epithelial malignancy; one of the most common forms of prostate cancer.

adjuvant therapy: treatment that is given after definitive therapy in the hope of preventing recurrence.

adrenal glands: bilateral glands situated above the kidneys. They produce certain hormones, both steroid and nonsteroid.

Ampicillin: an antibiotic; a penicillin derivative.

androgens: steroid hormones with properties of stimulating secondary male characteristics. They're produced primarily in the testicles, but also in the adrenal cortex.

antiandrogens: drugs that suppress or block the production of androgens.

antioxidant: a compound, such as a vitamin, that enables cells to recover from oxidated reactions by being scavengers of free radicals.

Anusol: a hydrogenated base used in the treatment of hemorrhoids.

Anusol HC: a similar compound, but with the addition of hydrocortisone to relieve inflammation.

barium drink: barium is an element that is radiographically opaque and can be used to identify viscous structures in the body. For example, a barium drink can identify the esophagus, the stomach, and small intestines.

basal cell carcinoma: a skin cancer. It can be locally invasive and recurrent, but generally does not metastasize (spread).

benign: describes the behavior of cells that lack the ability to invade adjacent tissue and metastasize.

bladder: an organ in which urine is collected. Its contraction causes urination.

bladder cystoscopy: visualization of the inside of the bladder by means of a scope inserted through the penis and urethra.

biopsy: obtainment of one or more specimens of tissue for histologic evaluation with the use of a microscope.

body cast: a synthetic polymer that creates a mode around the patient, in which a particular body position can be sustained.

bone scan: a radiographic evaluation that may demonstrate areas of increased bone activity. Such activity may represent metastatic disease, and/or arthritic changes, or fractures.

BPH: benign prostatic hypertropy (enlargement).

cancer: a term that describes certain groups of cells whose growth is no longer inhibited in a normal way, and which can spread throughout the body.

carcinoma: a malignant tumor of epithelial origin.

CAT scan: computer-assisted tomography. An image of a cross-section of the body or of certain organs, obtained by the use of low-energy X rays in conjunction with a computer.

catheter: a hollow tube that can be inserted in an orifice, usually through the urethra and into the bladder.

catheterization: the process of inserting a catheter.

CBC: complete blood count; a blood test that checks various blood cells.

Cerrobend: an alloy of lead, cadmium, bismuth and possibly some other metals.

chemotherapy: the use of certain drugs to kill malignant cells selectively.

CIEP: immunoassay, or electrophoresis; a test.

Cipro: an antibiotic used for a number of infections, particularly urinary tract infections.

conedown field: a smaller field than the standard field used in radiation therapy.

cryosurgery: the freezing of inner tissues, accomplishing goals similar to those of surgery; destruction of prostate cancer and benign cells by freezing.

CT scan: computerized tomography scan.

cysto-prostatitis: an inflammation of the bladder and the prostate gland, either infectious or noninfectious.

cystoscope: an instrument used to look at the bladder via the urethra.

Demerol: a narcotic analgesic (pain killer) given by injection.

digital: short for digital rectal exam.

dosimetrist: a trained technologist who helps formulate a treatment plan, often under the supervision of a medical physicist.

DRE: digital rectal exam.

dry orgasm: an orgasm without any ejaculate.

EIA: enzyme immunoassay; a test. The normal range is 0.0 to 2.5.

Empirin #3: Empirin (an analgesic) containing codeine.

ER: emergency room.

Erythromycin: an antibiotic effective against numerous organisms; it can be given orally or intravenously.

Eulexin: flutamide; a drug used in hormone treatment.

external-beam radiation: in contradistinction to an implant, internal radiation.

Flexeril: cyclobenzaprine; a muscle relaxant.

Floxin: a potent antibiotic commonly used for urinary tract infections.

flutamide: brand name: Eulexin.

gamma rays: X rays emitted by the decay of a radioactive nucleus.

Geocillin: an antibiotic.

Gleason score, or number, or grade: a pathologic determination predicting the rate of aggressiveness of a tumor, based on how it looks under a microscope. A prostate cancer is given a major pattern grade and a minor pattern grade, each from 1 to 5. When added together, the result is a Gleason score, which may range from 2 to 10.

gray: one gray is equivalent to 100 rads.

Halcion: a sleeping pill.

hc suppositories: suppositories containing hydrocortisone; they help shrink internal rectal tissues.

HIV: human immunodeficiency virus; a retrovirus that causes AIDS.

Hodgkin's disease: a type of lymphoma. This tumor is highly sensitive to both chemotherapy and radiation therapy.

hormone: a chemical, produced in one area of the body, that by means of the bloodstream can influence the metabolism of other tissues and organs.

hormone therapy: suppression of hormones as a means of achieving a specific result. In prostate cancer it is medication that suppresses androgens.

Imodium: a drug used to stop diarrhea.

impotence: inability to achieve and maintain an erection sufficient for intercourse.

incontinence: inability to maintain complete voluntary control over bladder or rectum.

interstitial radiation: irradiating tissues by means of radioactive sources that are placed either temporarily or permanently within the tissues.

IV: intravenous.

IVP: intravenous polygram.

linac: short for linear accelerator.

linear accelerator: the machine by which high-energy X rays are produced.

Lupron: leuprolide; a drug used to suppress the production of testosterone.

lymph node: a small gland housing lymphocytes. Such nodes are one of the first areas to fight infections, and one of the first to which cancers are spread.

lymphoma: a type of malignancy.

Macrodantin: an antibiotic that is very effective in urinary tract infections.

male hormones: hormones produced by the testicles and the adrenal glands.

malignant: describing the potential for cells to grow in an uncontrolled fashion and to spread to other areas the body.

mammogram: an X ray of the female breast, used for detecting an early stage of breast cancer.

mastectomy: surgical removal of the female breast.

melanoma: often a dangerous form of skin cancer, with a tendency to spread.

metastasis: the spread of a malignant tumor to other parts of the body.

monitor units: units of the amount of radiation administered.

morbidity: side effects or complications from a certain form of therapy.

morphine: a potent narcotic analgesic (sleep-inducing painkiller). It can be given orally, or injected into muscles or veins.

MRI: magnetic resonance imaging. A method of viewing cross-sections of the human body by using magnetic fields together with a computer. It does not use X rays.

needle biopsy: the process by which a needle is used to obtain tissue for histologic (cellular) diagnosis.

Noroxin: an antibiotic, often used in urinary tract infections.

oncogene: a gene that encourages the onset and growth of certain cancerous tumors.

oncologist: a physician who studies cancer and treats cancer patients.

orchiectomy: surgical removal of testicles.

PAP (prostatic acid phosphatase): the same as acid phosphatase or serum acid phosphatase.

pathologist: a physician who studies the effect of disease on tissues; who examines and evaluates biopsy specimens under the microscope.

Percocet: a narcotic painkiller.

perineal: relating to the area of the body that includes the genitalia.

planning session: one in which the radiation oncologist maps out the coordinates for radiation therapy.

Proctofoam: a drug used to soothe and shrink inflamed rectal tissues.

prostatitis: an inflammation (infectious or noninfectious) of the prostate gland.

PSA (prostate-specific antigen): a blood test of a specific cellular antigen produced by prostate cells or prostate cancer. The normal range is 1 to 4.

PSA density: PSA value over the volume of the prostate gland. It helps to predict for relative risk of cancer being present.

Pyridium: a drug, given orally, used to help eliminate the symptoms of bladder irritation. It turns urine a bright orange color.

rad: radiation absorbed dose.

radiation field: the area being treated by external-beam radiation.

radiation oncologist: a physician who supervises the use of radiation in the treatment of cancer patients.

radiation physicist: a physicist who works with the radiation oncologist to calculate and plan the radiation dose to be given. He also supervises the maintenance of the linear accelerator.

radiation therapist: a technologist who treats patients by means of radiation therapy.

radical prostatectomy: surgical removal of the prostate gland, sometimes including nearby lymph nodes.

remission: a state in which cancer has been removed.

retrograde ejaculation: ejaculation into the bladder upon orgasm.

retropubic prostatectomy: abdominal removal of the prostate; as distinguished from a perineal prostatectomy, which is done via the perineum.

self-injection method: used in impotence; injection into the base of the penis of a drug that helps achieve erection.

seminal vesicle: a pair of glands, on top of the prostate gland, that produce seminal fluid.

serum acid phosphatase: a blood test. The normal range is 0.0 to 2.0.

side effects: reaction of tissues to radiation therapy for prostate cancer; for example, more frequent urination, and discomfort on urinating, as a result of irritation of the bladder.

sonogram: an image created by the use of an ultrasound machine. An ultrasound machine uses the echoes of sound waves, in conjunction with a computer, to create images of organs inside the body.

squamous cell carcinoma: a type of skin cancer.

stage: the extent of a patient's disease.

staging: the process by which a patient's stage is determined.

strontium 89: a radioactive nucleid that can be incorporated into bone metastases; a suspended form of radiation therapy.

Temazepam: a sleeping pill.

testosterone: a hormone produced in the testicles.

Tetracycline: an antibiotic.

transrectal ultrasound: an ultrasound done via the rectum.

treatment room: the room, heavily lead-lined, in which the linear accelerator is housed, and where patients receive their radiation therapy.

TRUS: transrectal ultrasound.

tumor: a growth; it may be either benign or malignant.

TURP: transurethral resection of the prostate.

urine cytology: an examination of urine cells to check for the possibility of bladder malignancy.

vacuum method: a method, used in impotence, of achieving an erection.

watchful waiting: a philosophical approach to treating early-stage prostate cancer.

X-ray therapy: the use of high-energy photons in the treatment of conditions that are usually malignant but may also be benign.

Xylocaine: a numbing, painkilling medicine, given orally, or by IV injection, or by injection under the skin.

About the Author

Charles Neider has lived an adventurer's life. His five-decade career as a celebrated writer and photographer has taken him to diverse locations, from the cramped quarters of a Navy submarine, engaged in diving exercises in the North Atlantic, to the harsh, desolate Antarctic continent. A three-time Antarctic explorer, Neider survived a near-fatal helicopter crash that left him and three ill-equipped companions stranded at 12,250 feet on the slope on Mount Erebus (one of the world's few volcanoes with a lava lake) in temperatures of -31 degrees Fahrenheit. He has recounted his Antarctic experiences in the nonfiction works *Edge of the World: Ross Island, Antarctica* and *Beyond Cape Horn: Travels in the Antarctic.*

His passion for the adventurer's life and for the natural world has resulted in such anthologies as *Antarctica: Firsthand Accounts of Exploration and Endurance; Man against Nature: Firsthand Accounts of Adventure and Exploration; Great Shipwrecks and Castaways: Firsthand Accounts of Disasters at Sea; The Great West: A Treasury of Firsthand Accounts;* and *The Fabulous Insects: Essays by the Foremost Nature Writers.*

A writer's writer, Neider is the author of the novels *The White Citadel, Naked Eye, The Authentic Death of Hendry Jones* (filmed as *One-Eyed Jacks* produced, directed by, and starring Marlon Brando), *Overflight, Mozart and the Archbooby,* and *A Visit to*

Yazoo. His most recent fiction, *The Grotto Berg: Two Novellas*, has been hailed for being "reminiscent of Conrad" (*Publishers Weekly*) and "incredibly vivid, distinct, and compelling" (*Library Journal*). His work has been praised by the likes of Aldous Huxley, Saul Bellow, Thomas Mann, E. M. Forster, Marianne Moore, Max Eastman, Mark Schorer, Norman Cousins, William F. Buckley Jr., Alfred Kazin, Edmund Fuller, and even Albert Einstein.

As a literary critic he is the author of the seminal Kafka study, *The Frozen Sea*, and editor of *Tolstoy: Tales of Courage and Conflict*; *The Complete Short Stories of Washington Irving*; *The Stature of Thomas Mann*; *The Complete Short Stories of Robert Louis Stevenson*; *Essays of the Masters*; *Short Novels of the Masters*; *Great Short Stories of the Masters*; and a one-volume abridgment of Washington Irving's *George Washington: A Biography*.

A renowned Mark Twain scholar, he has edited such popular and enduring Twain collections as *The Complete Stories of Mark Twain*; *The Complete Essays of Mark Twain*; *The Complete Humorous Tales and Sketches of Mark Twain*; *The Selected Letters of Mark Twain*; *The Travels of Mark Twain*; *Life as I Find It: A Treasury of Mark Twain Rarities*; *Mark Twain: Plymouth Rock & the Pilgrims and Other Speeches*; *The Comic Mark Twain Reader*; and *Mark Twain's The Adventures of Colonel Sellers*.

Neider's remarkable photography of the vast Antarctic landscape and of stunning magnifications of minute aspects of gemstones has earned him wide acclaim.

He resides in Princeton, New Jersey, with his wife, Joan, a Thomas Mann scholar.